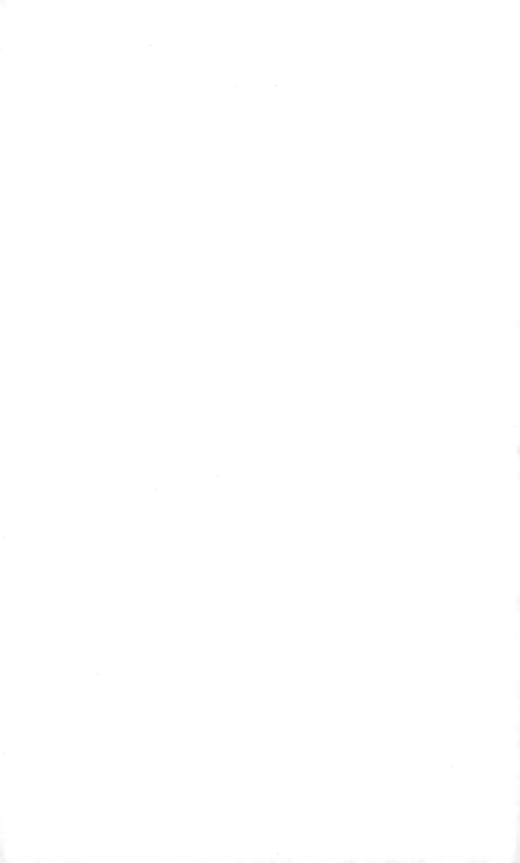

Pediatric Speech and Language: Perspectives on Interprofessional Practice

Editor

BRIAN B. SHULMAN

PEDIATRIC CLINICS
OF NORTH AMERICA

www.pediatric.theclinics.com

Consulting Editor
BONITA F. STANTON DISCARD

February 2018 • Volume 65 • Number 1

ELSEVIER

1600 John F. Kennedy Boulevard • Suite 1800 • Philadelphia, Pennsylvania, 19103-2899

http://www.theclinics.com

THE PEDIATRIC CLINICS OF NORTH AMERICA Volume 65, Number 1
February 2018 ISSN 0031-3955, ISBN-13: 978-0-323-56998-9

Editor: Kerry Holland
Developmental Editor: Casey Potter

The Pediatric Clinics of North America (ISSN 0031-3955) is published bimonthly by Elsevier Inc., 360 Park Avenue South, New York, NY 10010-1710. Months of issue are February, April, June, August, October, and December. Periodicals postage paid at New York, NY and additional mailing offices. Subscription prices are $216.00 per year (US individuals), $613.00 per year (US institutions), $292.00 per year (Canadian individuals), $816.00 per year (Canadian institutions), $338.00 per year (international individuals), $816.00 per year (international institutions), $100.00 per year (US students and residents), and $165.00 per year (international and Canadian residents and students). To receive students/resident rare, orders must be accompanied by name of affiliated institution, date of term, and the signature of program/residency coordinator on institution letterhead. Orders will be billed at individual rate until proof of status is received. Foreign air speed delivery is included in all Clinics subscription prices. All prices are subject to change without notice. **POSTMASTER:** Send address changes to The Pediatric Clinics of North America, Elsevier Health Sciences Division, Subscription Customer Service, 3251 Riverport Lane, Maryland Heights, MO 63043. **Customer Service: 1-800-654-2452 (US and Canada). From outside of the US and Canada: 1-314-447-8871. Fax: 1-314-447-8029. For print support, E-mail: JournalsCustomerService-usa@elsevier.com. For online support, E-mail: JournalsOnlineSupport-usa@elsevier.com.**

Reprints. For copies of 100 or more, of articles in this publication, please contact the Commercial Reprints Department, Elsevier Inc., 360 Park Avenue South, New York, NY 10010-1710. Tel.: 212-633-3874; Fax: 212-633-3820; E-mail: reprints@elsevier.com.

The Pediatric Clinics of North America is also published in Spanish by McGraw-Hill Inter-americana Editores S.A., Mexico City, Mexico; in Portuguese by Riechmann and Affonso Editores, Rua Comandante Coelho 1085, CEP 21250, Rio de Janeiro, Brazil; and in Greek by Althayia SA, Athens, Greece.

The Pediatric Clinics of North America is covered in MEDLINE/PubMed (Index Medicus), Excerpta Medica, Current Contents, Current Contents/Clinical Medicine, Science Citation Index, ASCA, ISI/BIOMED, and BIOSIS.

Printed in the United States of America.

PROGRAM OBJECTIVE
The goal of the *Pediatric Clinics of North America* is to keep practicing physicians and residents up to date with current clinical practice in pediatrics by providing timely articles reviewing the state-of-the-art in patient care.

TARGET AUDIENCE
All practicing pediatricians, physicians and healthcare professionals who provide patient care to pediatric patients.

LEARNING OBJECTIVES
Upon completion of this activity, participants will be able to:
1. Review concepts in interprofessional collaborative practice.
2. Discuss speech language care in pre-term and high-risk infants.
3. Recognize family-driven techniques in managing communication and language disorders.

ACCREDITATION
The Elsevier Office of Continuing Medical Education (EOCME) is accredited by the Accreditation Council for Continuing Medical Education (ACCME) to provide continuing medical education for physicians.

The EOCME designates this enduring material for a maximum of 15 *AMA PRA Category 1 Credit*(s)™. Physicians should claim only the credit commensurate with the extent of their participation in the activity.

All other healthcare professionals requesting continuing education credit for this enduring material will be issued a certificate of participation.

DISCLOSURE OF CONFLICTS OF INTEREST
The EOCME assesses conflict of interest with its instructors, faculty, planners, and other individuals who are in a position to control the content of CME activities. All relevant conflicts of interest that are identified are thoroughly vetted by EOCME for fair balance, scientific objectivity, and patient care recommendations. EOCME is committed to providing its learners with CME activities that promote improvements or quality in healthcare and not a specific proprietary business or a commercial interest.

The planning committee, staff, authors and editors listed below have identified no financial relationships or relationships to products or devices they or their spouse/life partner have with commercial interest related to the content of this CME activity:
Debra Anderson, MS, CCC-SLP; Kathleen C. Borowitz, MS, CCC-SLP; Stephen M. Borowitz, MD; Kathy L. Coufal, PhD; Laura M. Doss, DDS; Alan W. Dow, MD, MSHA; Anjali Fortna; Frank D. Golom, PhD; Kerry Holland; Randye F. Huron, MS, MD; Carole K. Ivey, PhD, OTR/L; Hildy S. Lipner, MA, CCC/SLP; Xueman Lucy Liu, AuD/CCC-A/FAAA, MS/CCC-SLP; Leah Logan; Sahira Long, MD, IBCLC, FAAP, FABM; Lemmietta G. McNeilly, PhD; Marie-Christine Potvin, PhD, OTR/L; Patricia A. Prelock, PhD, CCC-SLP, BCS-CL; Tommie L. Robinson Jr, PhD, CCC-SLP; Janet Simone Schreck, PhD; Mona M. Sedrak, PhD, PA; Mark D. Simms, MD, MPH; Nina Capone Capone Singleton, PhD, CCC-SLP; Bonita F. Stanton, MD; Carol A. Ukstins, MS, CCC/A, FAAA; Vignesh Viswanathan; Deborah R. Welling, AuD, CCC/A, FAAA; Julian L. Woods, PhD; Dawn M. Zhart, PhD.

The planning committee, staff, authors and editors listed below have identified financial relationships or relationships to products or devices they or their spouse/life partner have with commercial interest related to the content of this CME activity:
Ann W. Kummer, PhD, FASHA receives royalties/patents from Cengage; Jones & Bartlett Learning; and Super Duper® Publications.
Liliane Savard, PT, DPT, PCS receives royalties/patents from MedBridge Inc.
Brian B. Shulman, PhD, CCC-SLP, ASHA Fellow, BCS-CL, FASAHP receives royalties/patents from Jones & Bartlett Learning.

UNAPPROVED/OFF-LABEL USE DISCLOSURE
The EOCME requires CME faculty to disclose to the participants:
1. When products or procedures being discussed are off-label, unlabelled, experimental, and/or investigational (not US Food and Drug Administration [FDA] approved); and
2. Any limitations on the information presented, such as data that are preliminary or that represent ongoing research, interim analyses, and/or unsupported opinions. Faculty may discuss information about pharmaceutical agents that is outside of FDA-approved labelling. This information is intended solely for CME

and is not intended to promote off-label use of these medications. If you have any questions, contact the medical affairs department of the manufacturer for the most recent prescribing information.

TO ENROLL
To enroll in the *Pediatric Clinics of North America* Continuing Medical Education program, call customer service at 1-800-654-2452 or sign up online at http://www.theclinics.com/home/cme. The CME program is available to subscribers for an additional annual fee of USD 290.

METHOD OF PARTICIPATION
In order to claim credit, participants must complete the following:
1. Complete enrolment as indicated above.
2. Read the activity.
3. Complete the CME Test and Evaluation. Participants must achieve a score of 70% on the test. All CME Tests and Evaluations must be completed online.

CME INQUIRIES/SPECIAL NEEDS
For all CME inquiries or special needs, please contact elsevierCME@elsevier.com.

Contributors

CONSULTING EDITOR

BONITA F. STANTON, MD
Founding Dean, School of Medicine, Professor of Pediatrics, Seton Hall-Hackensack Meridian School of Medicine University, South Orange, New Jersey

EDITOR

BRIAN B. SHULMAN, PhD, CCC-SLP, ASHA Fellow, BCS-CL, FASAHP, FNAP
Dean and Professor of Speech-Language Pathology, School of Health and Medical Sciences, Professor of Pediatrics, Seton Hall-Hackensack Meridian School of Medicine, Seton Hall University, South Orange, New Jersey

AUTHORS

DEBRA ANDERSON, MS, CCC-SLP
Children's National Health System, Washington, DC

KATHLEEN C. BOROWITZ, MS, CCC-SLP
Department of Therapy Services, University of Virginia Health System, Charlottesville, Virginia

STEPHEN M. BOROWITZ, MD
Division of Pediatric Gastroenterology, Hepatology and Nutrition, University of Virginia, Charlottesville, Virginia

NINA CAPONE SINGLETON, PhD, CCC-SLP
Department of Speech-Language Pathology, School of Health and Medical Sciences, Seton Hall University, South Orange, New Jersey

KATHY L. COUFAL, PhD
Professor, Communication Disorders, University of Nebraska Omaha, Omaha, Nebraska

LAURA M. DOSS, DDS
Elizabeth Mueller and Associates, The Pediatric Dental Center, Mason, Ohio

ALAN W. DOW, MD, MSHA
Ruth and Seymour Perlin Professor of Internal Medicine and Health Administration, Assistant Vice President of Health Sciences, Interprofessional Education and Collaborative Care, Virginia Commonwealth University, Richmond, Virginia

FRANK D. GOLOM, PhD
Assistant Professor of Applied Psychology, Loyola University Maryland, Baltimore, Maryland

RANDYE F. HURON, MS, MD
Chief, Developmental and Behavioral Pediatrics, Director, Institute for Child Development, Joseph M. Sanzari Children's Hospital, Hackensack University Medical Center, Hackensack, New Jersey

CAROLE K. IVEY, PhD, OTR/L
Assistant Professor of Occupational Therapy, Virginia Commonwealth University, Richmond, Virginia

ANN W. KUMMER, PhD, FASHA
Senior Director, Division of Speech-Language Pathology, Cincinnati Children's Hospital Medical Center, Professor of Clinical Pediatrics and Otolaryngology, University of Cincinnati College of Medicine, Cincinnati, Ohio

HILDY S. LIPNER, MA, CCC/SLP
Chief, Pediatric Speech Pathology, Institute for Child Development, Joseph M. Sanzari Children's Hospital, Hackensack University Medical Center, Hackensack, New Jersey

XUEMAN LUCY LIU, AuD/CCC-A/FAAA, MS/CCC-SLP
Bethel Hearing and Speaking Training Center Inc., Corinth, Texas

SAHIRA LONG, MD, IBCLC, FAAP, FABM
Children's National Health System, School of Medicine & Health Sciences, The George Washington University, Washington, DC

LEMMIETTA G. McNEILLY, PhD
Chief Staff Officer, Speech-Language Pathology, American Speech-Language-Hearing Association, Rockville, Maryland

MARIE-CHRISTINE POTVIN, PhD, OTR/L
Associate Director, Clinical OTD Program, Associate Professor of Occupational Therapy, Philadelphia University, Philadelphia, Pennsylvania

PATRICIA A. PRELOCK, PhD, CCC-SLP, BCS-CL
Professor and Dean, College of Nursing and Health Sciences, The University of Vermont, Burlington, Vermont

TOMMIE L. ROBINSON Jr, PhD, CCC-SLP
Children's National Health System, Scottish Rite Center Childhood Language Disorders, School of Medicine & Health Sciences, The George Washington University, Washington, DC

LILIANE SAVARD, PT, DPT, PCS
Doctoral Student and Clinician at Zippy Life Physical Therapy, The University of Vermont, Vermont

JANET SIMON SCHRECK, PhD
Assistant Vice Provost for Education, Johns Hopkins University, Baltimore, Maryland

MONA M. SEDRAK, PhD, PA
Senior Associate Dean for Academic Affairs, School of Health and Medical Sciences, Seton Hall University, South Orange, New Jersey

BRIAN B. SHULMAN, PhD, CCC-SLP, ASHA Fellow, BCS-CL, FASAHP, FNAP
Dean and Professor of Speech-Language Pathology, School of Health and Medical Sciences, Professor of Pediatrics, Seton Hall-Hackensack Meridian School of Medicine, Seton Hall University, South Orange, New Jersey

MARK D. SIMMS, MD, MPH
Professor, Department of Pediatrics, Section of Developmental Pediatrics, Medical College of Wisconsin, Milwaukee, Wisconsin; Child Development Center, Children's Hospital of Wisconsin, Brookfield, Wisconsin

CAROL A. UKSTINS, MS, CCC/A, FAAA
Educational Audiologist, Newark Public Schools, Office of Special Education, Newark, New Jersey

DEBORAH R. WELLING, AuD, CCC/A, FAAA
Associate Professor and Director of Clinical Education, Seton Hall University, South Orange, New Jersey

JULIANN J. WOODS, PhD
Professor, School of Communication Science & Disorders, Florida State University, Tallahassee, Florida

DAWN M. ZAHRT, PhD
Associate Professor, Department of Pediatrics, Section of Developmental Pediatrics, Medical College of Wisconsin, Milwaukee, Wisconsin; Child Development Center, Children's Hospital of Wisconsin, Brookfield, Wisconsin

Contents

> Interprofessional collaborative practice (IPCP) is a service delivery approach
> that seeks to improve health care outcomes and the patient experience while
> simultaneously decreasing health care costs. This article reviews the core
> competencies and current trends associated with IPCP, including challenges
> faced by health care practitioners when working on interprofessional teams.
> Several conceptual frameworks and empirically supported interventions
> from the fields of organizational psychology and organization development
> are presented to assist health care professionals in transitioning their teams
> to a more interprofessionally collaborative, team-based model of practice.

> From a speech-language pathology perspective, there is a gap in interpro-
> fessional education/practice (IPE/IPP) that leads to a wait-and-see approach
> with late talkers (LTs). In line with the American Speech-Language-Hearing
> Association's *Strategic Pathway to Excellence*, this article attempts to bridge
> the gap, reexamining the panoptic view that most LTs "catch up" to their
> peers. The LTs who persist with language disorder should not be overlooked.
> Late talking can affect socialization and school readiness and can place
> some toddlers at risk for lifelong disability. Each state's early intervention
> program has an established IPP infrastructure. Parent-implemented inter-
> vention addresses risks and maximizes protective factors.

 Video content accompanies this article at http://www.pediatric.
theclinics.com.

> This article describes how different types of clefts affect the child's function
> and, in particular, the child's communication abilities. This article also de-
> scribes the evaluation process and various options for the treatment of
> affected speech. Because these children have many complicated needs
> over their entire growth period, it is important that they are referred by the pedi-
> atrician to a cleft palate/craniofacial team for the best care and best ultimate
> outcomes.

This article describes the Coaching in Context (CinC) process, a family-driven, culturally responsive structure that facilitates family identification and achievement of goals. CinC focuses on modification of the demands of an activity with guidance from a health care professional who coaches the family to increase their participation in everyday activities. An interprofessional team is key in this process. Working as a team and communicating effectively across professions supports the health professional who serves as the coach. Effective interprofessional team collaboration is possible; health professions share values for the delivery of the highest quality of care.

Feeding problems in infants and young children are common. In healthy children who are developing and growing normally, feeding problems are usually not serious and can be managed conservatively by reassuring the family and providing them with anticipatory guidance and follow-up. Most serious childhood feeding problems occur in children who have other medical, developmental, or behavioral problems. These are best evaluated and treated by an interprofessional team that can identify and address issues in the medical and/or developmental history, problems with oral motor control and function, problems with swallowing, and behavioral and/or sensory issues that may interfere with normal feeding.

The ability to communicate effectively with others is central to children's development. Delays or disruptions due to isolated expressive language delay, articulation errors, multiple sound production errors with motor planning deficits, or mixed expressive and receptive language delay often bring widespread consequences. Physical anomalies, neurologic and genetic disorders, cognitive and intellectual disabilities, and emotional disturbances may affect speech and language development. Communication disorders may be misdiagnosed as intellectual impairment or autism. Interdisciplinary evaluation should include speech and language assessment, physical and neurologic status, cognitive and emotional profile, and family and social history. This article describes assessment and reviews common pediatric communication disorders.

Dental caries is the single most common chronic disease of childhood in the United States. Access to dental care is one of the barriers to improved oral health for children. Primary care providers who routinely treat children have an established role in the prevention and early identification of health problems; thus, they are ideal front-line providers who can detect oral health discrepancies and begin the process of care and prevention.

Otitis Media: Beyond the Examining Room   105

Deborah R. Welling and Carol A. Ukstins

The management of hearing loss associated with otitis media is multifaceted. Clinical practice guidelines set the collaborative prescriptive standards for the medical management of otitis media in children. Treatment of this condition does not end with the medical practitioner. There are far-reaching effects of otitis media and its sequelae that permeate every aspect of patients' lives, including physiologic, educational, and psychosocial. Therefore, a comprehensive interprofessional treatment plan must be designed taking into consideration best practices from a range of professions to maximize clinical outcomes, including the treating physician, speech-language pathologist, clinical audiologist, educational audiologist, and professionals in the educational setting.

Using the International Classification of Functioning, Disability and Health Framework to Achieve Interprofessional Functional Outcomes for Young Children: A Speech-Language Pathology Perspective   125

Lemmietta G. McNeilly

The International Classification of Functioning, Disability and Health framework is an excellent tool to facilitate the writing of functional goals for children who exhibit communication disorders and other developmental problems that require services from professionals in multiple therapeutic areas. The holistic view of children provides each professional with an approach that integrates how one's specific health conditions and contextual factors influence a child's functioning and participation in daily activities. This allows the interprofessional team to view the child as a person, recognizing how one need influences another within his or her environment.

Developmental and Interprofessional Care of the Preterm Infant: Neonatal Intensive Care Unit Through High-Risk Infant Follow-up   135

Hildy S. Lipner and Randye F. Huron

Practices in the neonatal intensive care unit (NICU) that reduce infant stress and respond to behavioral cues positively influence developmental outcomes. Proactive developmental surveillance and timely introduction of early intervention services improve outcomes for premature infants. A model that emphasizes infant development and a continuum of care beginning in the NICU with transition to outpatient monitoring and provision of early intervention services is hypothesized to support the most optimal outcomes for premature infants.

Interprofessional Collaborative Practice in Early Intervention   143

Kathy L. Coufal and Juliann J. Woods

Professionals in pediatric practice encounter infants and toddlers with developmental delays, disabilities, or complex chronic health conditions

PEDIATRIC CLINICS OF NORTH AMERICA

Foreword

Pediatric Speech and Language: Perspectives on Interprofessional Practice

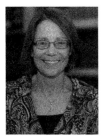

Bonita F. Stanton, MD
Consulting Editor

Despite all of the advances that have been made in the broad field of communications over the last several decades, much of an individual's ability to transmit information and emotions remains tied to his or her facility with speech. At any given point of time, an estimated six million children less than 18 years of age are experiencing a speech or language disorder. One in every ten Americans, across all ages, races, and genders, has experienced or currently lives with some type of speech, language, or communication disorder.[1]

The first few years of life represent a critical period for speech and language development. Children who do not use language normally from birth through early childhood may fail to fully develop language skills. Approximately 5% of children in first grade have identifiable speech impairments; with advancing age, some of these disorders will decline (such as stuttering), with higher rates persisting among boys compared to girls.[1,2]

Speech impairments arise from myriad conditions: hearing loss; developmental, psychiatric, and neurologic disorders; cognitive disorders; drug abuse; cleft lip or palate; and emotional disorders, as well as many for which there are no identifiable explanations or causes. "Specific language impairments (SPL)" describe clinically significant impairments in a child's development of spoken language in the absence of identifiable sensory or neurodevelopmental disorders. Spoken language in this case includes the ability to understand words, sentences, and connected speech as well as the ability to express messages using appropriate vocabulary, grammar, and discourse. There appears to be great variability in prevalence of SPL because of definitional differences and the substantial but unpredictable recovery during the early preschool years, which flattens over time.[3,4]

Pediatr Clin N Am 65 (2018) xv–xvi
https://doi.org/10.1016/j.pcl.2017.10.002
0031-3955/18/© 2017 Published by Elsevier Inc.

The importance of speech and language disorders to children throughout their childhood and adulthood is in itself substantial reason for all pediatricians and child health workers to be interested in any updates on these disorders. But beyond the importance of this topic in general, this issue of *Pediatric Clinics of North America*, compiled by Brian Shulman and colleagues from a wide array of disciplines, is especially exciting because it focuses on advances that involve collaboration between multiple professions. The advances discussed herein generally required the collaboration of multiple disciplines, resulting in "interprofessional advances." Some of these advances result from new technologies emerging from the interprofessional collaboration; others emerged from the new application of existing technologies emerging from interprofessional consultation, and still others from borrowing therapeutic or diagnostic strategies from one field by a member of another field. What emerges is a rich and innovative path forward to minimizing or eliminating speech and language difficulties among children and yet another example of how much is to be gained by working across professions.

Bonita F. Stanton, MD
Seton Hall-Hackensack Meridian School of Medicine University
400 South Orange Avenue
South Orange, NJ 07079, USA

E-mail address:
bonita.stanton@shu.edu

REFERENCES

1. Available at: https://www.psychologytoday.com/conditions/communication-disorders. Accessed September 17, 2017.
2. Available at: https://www.nidcd.nih.gov/health/statistics/statistics-voice-speech-and-language. Accessed September 17, 2017.
3. Tomblin JB, Smith E, Zhang X. Epidemiology of specific language impairment: prenatal and perinatal risk factors. J Commun Disord 1997;30:325–44.
4. Law J, Boyle J, Harris F, et al. Prevalence and natural history of primary speech and language delay: findings from a systematic review of the literature. Int J Lang Commun Disord 2000;35:165–88.

Preface

Pediatric Speech and Language Perspectives on Interprofessional Practice

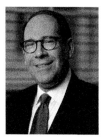

Brian B. Shulman, PhD, CCC-SLP, ASHA Fellow, BCS-CL, FASAHP, FNAP
Editor

Like many other medical and health-related professions, the speech-language pathology and audiology professions have been responding to the changes in the delivery of health care due to legislative and regulatory policy changes at the federal and state levels. To this end and as a result of reports from the World Health Organization[1–4] and the Institute of Medicine,[5–7] health care professionals are now addressing health care service delivery within an interprofessional, collaborative practice and patient outcomes context. This issue of *Pediatric Clinics of North America* presents articles that address clinical care to a variety of pediatric speech and language clinical populations. Each piece provides its own perspective on interprofessional care, while the first and last articles, respectively, introduce and then synthesize all of the articles into a cogent issue.

In their opening piece, Golom and Schreck take us on a journey through the "interprofessional practice world" addressing some of the strengths, barriers, and challenges we may face as we transition to an interprofessional perspective of care. Capone Singleton approaches interprofessional practice as it relates to the "wait-and-see" approach that some colleagues might espouse to when evaluating the speech and language development in young children. Kummer provides readers of this issue with an informative guide to an approach to assessing and treating children with cleft palate speech and velopharyngeal insufficiency from an interprofessional perspective, with this population of speech-impaired children. Prelock and colleagues from the University of Vermont share their interprofessional perspectives on working with children with autism and their families. The Borowitz and Borowitz article pairs a speech-language pathologist and a pediatric gastroenterologist in addressing

Pediatr Clin N Am 65 (2018) xvii–xix
https://doi.org/10.1016/j.pcl.2017.10.001   **pediatric.theclinics.com**
0031-3955/18/© 2017 Published by Elsevier Inc.

assessment and intervention for infants and children with feeding problems. Clearly, the collaboration between these two professions, at a minimum, reinforces the value of interprofessional care. The piece by Liu, Zhart, and Simms provides a comprehensive and interprofessional approach to developing differential diagnoses of children with a variety of communication disorders.

Recently, oral health has been at the forefront of concerns expressed by colleagues in pediatric dentistry and in speech-language pathology given its importance in the development of appropriate speech production. To that end, Sedrak and Doss describe an interprofessional approach to pediatric oral health. This issue continues with a discussion on otitis media by audiologists, Welling and Utskins, followed by McNeilly's application of the International Classification of Functioning, Disability, and Health[4] framework to achieve interprofessional outcomes for speech-language–impaired children. Speech-language pathologist, Lipner, and developmental pediatrician, Huron, describe their interprofessional approach to the developmental care of the preterm infant followed by high-risk infant follow-up at Hackensack University Medical Center. As speech and language–impaired children transition from infancy to the early childhood years, Coufal and Woods discuss how interprofessional practice and collaboration is a critical approach to providing early intervention. Children seen on an outpatient basis for speech and language assessment and intervention often encounter an interprofessional service delivery context. Robinson and his colleagues from the Children's National Health System in the District of Columbia describe the role of the speech-language pathologist within an ambulatory care clinic. As noted earlier, the final article by Dow, Ivey, and Shulman synthesizes a majority of the themes presented herein and also describes challenges and predictions for the future of pediatric speech-language pathology within an interprofessional care model.

Enjoy this issue!

Brian B. Shulman, PhD, CCC-SLP, ASHA Fellow, BCS-CL, FASAHP, FNAP
Office of the Dean
School of Health and Medical Sciences
Seton Hall University
400 South Orange Avenue, NJ 07079, USA

E-mail address:
brian.shulman@shu.edu

REFERENCES

1. World Health Organization (WHO). Interprofessional collaborative practice in primary health care: nursing and midwifery perspectives. Six case studies. Geneva (Switzerland): WHO; 2013.
2. World Health Organization (WHO). Transformative scale up of health professional education. Geneva (Switzerland): WHO; 2011.
3. World Health Organization (WHO). Framework for action on interprofessional education and collaborative practice. Geneva (Switzerland): WHO; 2010.
4. World Health Organization (WHO). The International Classification of Functioning, Disability and Health, Children and Youth version. Geneva (Switzerland): WHO; 2007. Available at: http://www.who.int/classifications/icf/en/. Accessed July 14, 2017.
5. Institute of Medicine (IOM). To err is human: building a safer health system. Washington, DC: National Academies Press; 2000.

6. Institute of Medicine (IOM). Crossing the quality chasm: a new health system for the 21st century. Washington, DC: National Academies Press; 2001.
7. Institute of Medicine (IOM). Measuring the impact of interprofessional education on collaborative practice and patient outcomes. Washington, DC: National Academies Press; 2015.

The Journey to Interprofessional Collaborative Practice

Are We There Yet?

Frank D. Golom, PhD[a], Janet Simon Schreck, PhD[b],*

KEYWORDS

- Interprofessional • Collaboration • Teams • Team building • Communication
- Health care • Organization development

KEY POINTS

- Interprofessional collaborative practice (IPCP) is an aspirational holistic approach to health care. Clinicians who seek to deliver IPCP must achieve core competencies related to teamwork and team effectiveness.
- Although there are a number of daunting systemic factors that are miring the journey to IPCP, clinicians should seek the knowledge and tools required to design effective collaboration.
- Frameworks from disciplines specifically devoted to the study of group and team dynamics, including organizational psychology and organization development, can assist clinicians on this journey.
- Organizational teams frequently act more like groups than actual teams, in part because they lack truly interdependent and shared work, collective accountability, and team member complementarity.
- Several strategies can improve team collaboration and functioning, including developing clear and challenging goals, clarifying team member roles/responsibilities, and reviewing all processes and procedures.

For decades, speech–language pathologists have worked alongside other health care professionals to provide care for children presenting with disorders of communication, cognition, and swallowing. Yet, evolving reimbursement models, increasingly complex diagnoses and intervention strategies, and greater calls for holistic approaches to

Disclosure Statement: F.D. Golom has no relevant disclosures to report. J.S. Schreck has no relevant disclosures to report.
[a] Department of Psychology, Loyola University Maryland, 4501 North Charles Street, Baltimore, MD 21210, USA; [b] The Johns Hopkins University, 3400, Office of the Provost, North Charles Street, Baltimore, MD 21218, USA
* Corresponding author.
E-mail address: jschreck@jhu.edu

Pediatr Clin N Am 65 (2018) 1–12
https://doi.org/10.1016/j.pcl.2017.08.017
pediatric.theclinics.com

patient care now necessitate professional interdependency in a way that transcends the "work alongside" approach.[1] Recognized by the American Speech-Language-Hearing Association as a model that is key to its *Envisioned Future* for speech–language pathologists,[2] interprofessional collaborative practice (IPCP) is a service delivery approach that seeks to improve health care outcomes and the patient experience while simultaneously decreasing health care cost. IPCP is a practice ideal that is intuitively appealing to clinicians and simultaneously challenging to achieve. This article defines IPCP and provides clinicians with tools and frameworks from the fields of organizational psychology and organization development that can be used to foster IPCP in practice settings.

DEFINING INTERPROFESSIONAL COLLABORATIVE PRACTICE

The World Health Organization[3] describes IPCP as the provision of comprehensive health services by multiple health workers from different professional backgrounds who seek to work with patients, families, caregivers, and communities to provide the highest quality of care across settings. This definition highlights multiple key aspects of IPCP in that it is patient and family centered, relationship focused, and community based. Interprofessional team-based care is further defined as care delivery by intentionally created, usually relatively small work groups, whose members recognize themselves as having both a collective identity and a shared responsibility for a patient or group of patients.[4] Clinicians who practice the IPCP model are engaged with each other, and with patients and their stakeholders, in a process-oriented and outcome-driven manner that is holistic, reflective, integrative, and cohesive.[5]

The movement toward IPCP has occurred in tandem with the emergence of interprofessional education (IPE). IPE occurs when "students from two or more professions learn about, from and with each other to enable effective collaboration and improve outcomes."[3] IPE, which has largely emerged from the fields of medicine, nursing, pharmacy and public health, is generally associated with preprofessional academic and clinical preparation that occurs in colleges and universities. IPE, however, can also be used in the continuing education setting as a means for training practicing clinicians in the IPCP model.[5]

When we present IPCP to experienced speech–language pathologists at national conferences, we often hear such proclamations as, "This is nothing new! I have been doing this my whole career," and "Multidisciplinary…interdisciplinary…interprofessional…it's just the new hot term for the same concept." Although it can be argued that IPCP evolved from multidisciplinary and interdisciplinary practice models that dominated the 1980s and 1990s, as shown in **Table 1**, interprofessional collaboration is distinctive from multidisciplinary and interdisciplinary approaches in its philosophy, structure, and process.[6] Interprofessional collaboration is a systems-focused approach that targets the provision of holistic care by team members with equal authority and shared responsibility and accountability.[7] To effectively practice IPCP, the clinician must intentionally seek to develop a number of interrelated professional competencies.

Interprofessional Collaborative Practice Core Competencies

In 2011, the Interprofessional Education Collaborative (IPEC)[8] published its core competencies for interprofessional collaborative practice. Synthesizing deliberations and recommendations of experts from 6 national health professions associations, the report delineated and defined the interprofessional foundational competencies required for future health professionals to deliver interprofessional collaborative care. In 2016, IPEC released an updated document that incorporated input from 9

Table 1
Differences between multidisciplinary, interdisciplinary and IPCP teams

Multidisciplinary Team	Interdisciplinary Teams	IPCP Teams
Hierarchical	Less hierarchical but not equal	No hierarchy or territory; all members are equal
Excludes the patient and family; patients and families are merely recipients of care	More inclusive of the patient and family; patients and families viewed as team members with less authority	Patient and family focused; patient and family are equally powerful team members
Strong leader gathers, synthesizes, disseminates data	Less dependent on a central team leader	No central leader; leadership is shared among team members
Members have limited knowledge of others' disciplines and roles	Members understand each others' disciplines and roles but operate within disciplinary boundaries	Role clarification is a conscious effort; input from other disciplines is intentionally sought
Members are accountable to self	Members are accountable to self and each other	Shared responsibility and accountability by the members of the team as well as the team as a unit
Limited communication between team members	More communication between team members, but often ineffective owing to time constraints, use of disciplinary jargon	Continuous, seamless, dynamic, effective communication among team members

Abbreviation: IPCP, interprofessional collaborative practice.

additional professions and broadened the interprofessional competencies to better achieve the World Health Organization triple aim of improving the patient care experience, improving the health of populations, and reducing the per capita cost of health care.[3,4] Endorsed by the American Speech-Language-Hearing Association in 2013[9] and depicted in **Fig. 1**, the core competencies include interprofessional communication practices, roles and responsibilities for collaborative practice, values and ethics for interprofessional practice, and interprofessional teamwork and team-based practice.

Applying the IPEC core competencies, we find that speech–language pathologists who choose to practice using the IPCP methodology must be interprofessional communicators who use communication tools and techniques that allow for respectful, clear, and effective communication with team members. They must be aware of common professional hierarchies that contribute to dysfunctional communication patterns and be routine givers and receivers of feedback regarding both individual and team performance and communication. Practicing IPCP also requires that clinicians place the interest of the patient at the center of service delivery and treat all members of the team, including the patient and family, with the mutual respect and trust reflective of an equal partnership. Effective IPCP practitioners must recognize their own roles and limitations and engage diverse professionals with complementary expertise to meet specific needs of patients and populations. They also must incorporate relationship-building values, effective team-building strategies, and self-reflection in their work as they engage other disciplines in shared patient-centered problem solving. Finally, practitioners engaging in IPCP must share accountability with their patients, their fellow professionals, and their communities for outcomes.

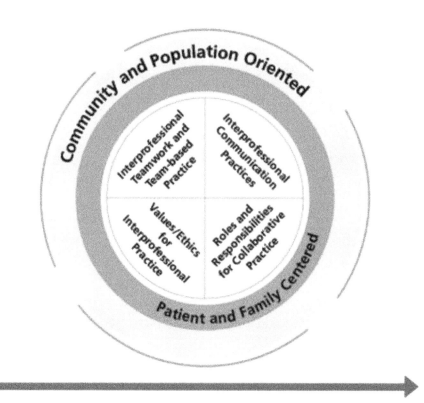

The Learning Continuum pre-licensure through practice trajectory

Fig. 1. Interprofessional collaboration competency domains. (*From* Interprofessional Education Expert Panel. Core competencies for interprofessional collaborative practice: 2016. Washington, DC: Interprofessional Education Collaborative; 2016; with permission.)

Is there anyone who truly practices this way? Do reimbursement models allow clinicians time to reflect on their communication and the effectiveness of the team? How many teams have truly achieved equitable roles among varying disciplines, patients, and families? Do clinicians really have the confidence to learn from others who may approach a problem differently than their preparation or experience? In many ways, the field of speech–language pathology is just beginning its journey to IPCP, a journey mired by daunting systemic forces, including dated clinical training models, archaic organizational hierarchies, and dysfunctional reimbursement systems. Although IPCP is intuitively attractive to clinicians, it remains an aspirational practice ideal that can only occur when there is both a team structure supportive of collaboration and a professional commitment to collaborative practice.[10] One way that speech–language pathologists can continue the movement toward IPCP is to more intentionally seek the requisite knowledge and tools required to design truly effective collaborative teams.

ORGANIZATIONAL FRAMEWORKS FOR FOSTERING INTERPROFESSIONAL COLLABORATIVE PRACTICE

Given the central role of effective teamwork in the latest IPEC competencies, the journey to IPCP runs, in part, through disciplines outside the health care arena, including those that specialize in the scientific study of group and team dynamics. To this end, the fields of organizational psychology, organizational behavior, and organization development may be helpful to those interested in enacting some of the core domains of IPCP, namely team functioning and role clarification. This section reviews some of the basic literature on groups and teams in organizational psychology, including several frameworks and intervention tools that can assist those interested in shifting their work toward a more interprofessionally driven space.

The Group Versus Team Distinction

The distinction between multidisciplinary/interdisciplinary practice and interprofessional collaboration (**Table 1**) finds an analog in the organizational literature and the distinction between groups and teams. Although not universally shared or agreed upon by organizational psychologists,[11] several have noted that the concepts of groups and teams may be conceptually distinct from each other along a number of focal areas.[12–14] For example, Katzenbach and Smith[13] note that groups and teams differ in terms of their accountability to the collective, the type of work they produce and the style of their interactions. Whereas teams and team members are generally accountable to each other, deliver a collective product that cannot be produced by any 1 member alone, and are composed of individuals with complementary skills, groups often require far less interdependent work, collective accountability, or complementarity. Group members may find themselves working next to each other based on related expertise or similar work assignments (eg, hospital or university department), but the degree of task interdependence that exists among them is relatively low; tasks can generally be completed, outcomes can be produced, and work can be organized with minimal input, discussion, and collaboration from other group members.[13]

For those who have followed the journey from multidisciplinary practice to true interprofessional collaboration, the distinction between groups and teams in the organizational literature may sound familiar. Multidisciplinary or even interdisciplinary work often involves working next to rather than working with, often as a result of low interdependence stemming from the absence of a true shared purpose or collective work product.[13,15] The group versus team distinction is not simply academic or pedantic; participants in executive education workshops we have facilitated find it to be practically resonant, likely because most of the lip service organizations devote to teams and teamwork is just that. Much of what we have labeled teamwork in modern organizational life actually involves working with others in configurations of pooled, rather than shared, activity,[11,16] potentially rendering practitioners unable to deliver on the promise of interprofessional practice despite decades of encouragement.[6]

Conditions for Team Effectiveness

A better understanding of teamwork, team building, and team effectiveness should assist health care practitioners on the journey to IPE and collaboration. There is an extensive literature detailing team effectiveness and its antecedents, with thousands of academic and popular articles written on the subject.[11] Hackman[15] defines effective teams as those that serve their clients, grow as a team, and contribute to individual team members' learning and well-being. Additionally, effectiveness is achieved more through the design of the team's collective work than through individual personality or leadership style. This emphasis on the task and structurally based drivers of team effectiveness is consistent with other common team building models in the organization development literature (eg, Burke[17]), and is easily transportable across a diverse array of contexts where interprofessional collaboration is required.

According to Hackman,[15] the most effective teams are those that are (1) "real," (2) have a compelling and aspiring direction for their work, and (3) have enabling structures that facilitate rather than interfere with the completion of interdependent team tasks. Similar to the group versus team distinction, the notion that effective teams need to be real teams addresses the fact that to function well, teams need to spring from a place of collaborative work rather than exist in name only. To that end, real teams are defined[15] as those that have an actual joint project on which to collaborate, clear boundaries that identify team members from nonmembers, delimited authority to make decisions about that collaboration, and some degree of membership stability over time. A well-defined team task is particularly essential to this endeavor. Much of the work teams are asked to do in organizations involves the coordination of individual contributions of input rather than delivering a product or service that no one person could produce alone. For this reason, clearly delineated interdependent tasks that are jointly understood by all members are essential to being able to work together in an interprofessional capacity, and are a prerequisite for team effectiveness.[11,15,18,19]

A clear and compelling direction for the team's work is also essential for effective functioning.[15] As Hackman notes,[15] teams require a direction or purpose that energizes, orients, and engages all members, whether that purpose is self-set by the members or imposed by someone in positional authority over the team. This notion of direction as a motivating and guiding force in organizational life is not new; numerous publications have discussed the importance of vision in the context of leadership, organizational strategy, and even individual executive development.[20] In the context of teamwork, however, a clear and challenging direction not only motivates team members, it often serves an important coordinating function by influencing other aspects of team decision making, including role assignments, task-related communication, and the selection of different task performance strategies.[11,15] Not surprisingly, establishing a team's direction vis-à-vis well-defined goals and objectives is a common feature of many popular team building programs, and is a tangible intervention that can be used to promote interprofessional practice in the health care arena.[21–23]

In addition to being a team in more than name only and having a clear and challenging direction for the work, effective teams are also structurally set up for success.[15] In fact, the structural antecedents of team effectiveness have been written about extensively in the organizational literature, and include such aspects of team composition as size, demographic and functional diversity, personality, values, and ability.[11] For example, team size is a significant predictor of effectiveness, with both process and performance deteriorating if the number of team members becomes too large. Although estimates on what constitutes too large vary by study, Hackman[15] argues that most project teams of greater than 5 or 6 will begin to suffer some form of process loss that may interfere with productivity. A certain amount of diversity seems to be essential for team functioning as well, particularly with respect to creativity and innovation, because research suggests that diverse teams demonstrate better problem solving and more creative solutions than homogenous teams,[24] particularly over time.[25] Other important aspects of structure that have received attention in the literature include the design of the work itself,[26] a clear understanding of team member roles,[27,28] and deliberately articulated norms related to task management and group procedures.[15] Similar to defining goals and objectives, attending to these additional structural aspects is often at the heart of diagnosing and ameliorating team-related performance challenges.[21]

Team Building Models and Approaches

The research findings on team effectiveness serve an important backdrop for understanding the conditions that foster productivity in work teams, but they are in and of themselves not always amenable to practical application. As a result, several team building models and approaches have been developed for organizational use over the years, including popular group-level interventions originating in the field of organization development.[23] The most common of these interventions is known as the Goals, Roles, Processes and Interpersonal relations (GRPI) model.[17]

The GRPI model of team building was originally developed by Beckhard[29] and has become well-regarded in the organization development field over the last several decades.[17,30,31] According to the model, conflictual and ineffective processes in teams can be attributed to a lack of clarity and understanding around goals and objectives (G), team member roles (R), processes and procedures for collaboration (P), and members' different interpersonal styles (I). To that end, team building using GRPI involves walking members through a number of activities aimed at clarifying and developing a shared understanding of the objectives, roles, and norms of conduct needed to guide the team back to effective functioning and productivity.

For example, if the team is early in its formation, or there is confusion around its objectives and priorities, a team building session using the GRPI model would focus on goal development and clarification so that member efforts are all moving in the same direction and toward the same end, consistent with Hackman's[15] notion of a clear and compelling direction. If goals and objectives are well-defined, then another GRPI-based intervention might focus on determining whether team members have a shared understanding of their own and each other's roles and responsibilities, particularly given the goals and priorities they have set out to accomplish.[17] If roles are clear, attention may then be paid to actively delineating operating procedures and processes, including norms of conduct, so that team members may again develop a shared understanding not only of what they are working on and who should be working on what, but also how and when they intend to accomplish that work. **Table 2** provides a description of common team building interventions related to goals, roles, processes and procedures, and interpersonal relations, including specific tools and strategies that can be used for each type of intervention.

There are several assumptions underneath the GRPI model that are important to note. First, organization development scholars have argued that the GRPI model can and should be used hierarchically.[17] That is, one should focus on processes and procedures only if goals and roles are clear and unambiguous. If goals and roles are not well-articulated or understood, then the focus of the team building intervention should begin with goal setting and clarification. The conceptual logic beneath this assertion is simply that ambiguity at one level often fuels symptomatic conflict at lower levels, and to remain focused at the lower level is to fail to address the root cause of the conflict.[17,31] Second, some organization development practitioners[31] believe that about 80% of conflict in groups can be attributed to not having clear goals and objectives, with the remaining 20% being due to role (13%) and process (6%) ambiguity, and, finally, poor interpersonal relations (1%). Taken together, these 2 assumptions are grounded in the belief that, although much of the attention in ineffective teams is devoted to problematic team members and their interpersonal conflicts with each other, the true causes of poor team dynamics are often upstream—contextual and structural. If the goal of team building is to produce sustainable, positive changes in group functioning and performance, then all interventions should be targeted

Table 2
GRPI model components, descriptions and sample interventions

Team Building Component	Description	Sample Interventions
Goals	Developing and clarifying both individual and team-based goals and objectives, often with some attention to the alignment between individual, team and organizational goals.	Goal development/alignment SMART goal planning
Roles	Developing a deeper and clearer understanding of the roles and responsibilities of each team member, including the degree of authority/responsibility granted to each role.	Role clarification exercise Responsibility charting
Processes and procedures (see Problem solving)	Discussing, identifying, and addressing processes and procedures that may be associated with task-related performance difficulties, including implicit norms or codes of conduct.	Before action and after action reviews Team self-correction training Process consultation
Interpersonal relations	Developing individual self-awareness and interpersonal skills related to effective team membership, including communication, trust, and conflict.	Personality assessments Individual coaching

Abbreviation: GRPI, goals, roles, processes and interpersonal relations.
Data from Refs.[15,17,21,22]

accordingly and avoid focusing on the individual level. As a result, we do not discuss individual or interpersonal interventions in this article in any depth.

Last, although empirical support for the assumptions beneath the GRPI model is lacking, metaanalytic reviews[22,23] of different team building interventions largely support the component pieces of the model and an overall approach to team building that helps "groups examine, diagnose and act upon their behavior."[22] An initial review of the team building literature found that of 4 possible classes of team building interventions (eg, goal setting, role clarification, problem solving, and interpersonal relations), only role clarification had a modest positive effect on both subjective and objective measures of team performance. However, this finding was replicated and expanded on in a more rigorous metaanalysis 10 years later.[22] In this study, all 4 components of team building were found to have an effect on affective, process, and performance outcomes. Additionally, goal setting ($\rho = .37$) and role clarification ($\rho = .35$) had the strongest impact, consistent with GRPI and its assumption that goal and role clarity exert the largest influences on group functioning. As the authors concluded, "all the components of team building had a moderate effect on outcomes but the Goal-Setting and Role Clarification components had the largest effect."[22]

Recommendations for Interprofessional Collaborative Practice

From an IPCP practice perspective, the implications of the team building research and the GRPI model are fairly clear. First, interprofessional teams in the health care arena that wish to function as real teams should spend considerable time seeking a shared understanding of their purpose and direction as well as clarity related to the specific tasks on which they may be working. In our experience consulting with professionals from a range of industries, this task is easier said than done. Interprofessional health care teams are likely composed of staff from disparate disciplines, training, and functional expertise. Each of these differences is likely to influence the way the team's purpose and specific tasks are framed. Physicians, psychologists, and speech–language pathologists may have different definitions of the problem space, and of success. To work together interprofessionally is to spend substantial time negotiating these differences in a deliberate and structured fashion, often via an explicit discussion of goals and priorities using widely available goal-setting tools (eg, SMART goals).[21] To that end, a focus on the actual needs of the patient rather than on disciplinary orthodoxy may be particularly useful in helping interprofessional teams to develop a shared understanding of their work.

A clear explication of the team's purpose and goals, particularly in patient-centered ways, should also have the added benefit of helping to clarify the specific roles that are needed to ensure goal attainment. More plainly stated, task clarity can drive all other decisions an interprofessional team might make, including who should be performing what responsibilities and when, and what additional resources and support structures may be necessary.[22] There are numerous tools in the organization development literature for addressing role clarity concerns, including structured role clarification exercises and responsibility charting (see Dyer and colleagues[21]). Role clarification exercises generally require all individuals on the team to come to a shared understanding of their own roles and the roles of each team member. Additionally, the process frequently allows members to have explicit conversations about what they need from the team and what the team can expect from them related to executing the role in question.[21] Responsibility charting[17,32] is another explicit intervention, forcing team members to discuss, for each task that needs to be completed, which members are responsible for completing the task, which members are ultimately accountable for the outcome, and which need only to be informed or consulted. In our experience, responsibility charting often encourages teams to confront some of the subtle yet powerful authority dynamics that are often at the heart of team-related performance difficulties, including discipline and rank hierarchies that likely exist under the surface of interprofessional health care teams.[33]

Although goal setting and role clarification are often sufficient for helping teams to improve their functioning and productivity,[22] there are occasions where more explicit and structured discussions around team norms, processes, and procedures are necessary.[15] There are several interventions for approaching such discussions and helping teams to problem solve, including structured before action and after action reviews[34] and team self-correction training,[35,36] as well as more open-ended general discussions regarding processes and procedures.[15,37] Regardless of the specific approach used, the important implication for IPCP is that an explicit discussion of team norms, codes of conduct, and dynamics is necessary for healthy group functioning and for the creation of shared mental models for working together.[11,15] Encouraging teams to make before action and after action reviews a regular practice and to build recurring process checks into their meetings may help both their learning and their ability to reflect on and change strategies as necessary. Although not exhaustive, Schein[37] discusses a number of important group process variables that are predictive of performance, including communication, conflict management and decision making. Encouraging interprofessional teams to clarify and develop a shared understanding of the acceptable and unacceptable behaviors associated with each of these processes is important for constructively navigating the coordination difficulties frequently associated with diverse health care professionals working together.

Concluding Thoughts: The Importance of Context

As any social scientist will tell you, context matters. A number of aspects of the industry and work environment are likely to impact the effectiveness of any team, even with the most deliberate of team building strategies and interventions. We are not oblivious to these larger systemic forces, and indeed believe the journey to true interprofessional collaboration has been hamstrung by the lack of alignment between the team-based competencies reviewed herein and industry practices, reimbursement and incentive structures, and outdated training programs. Nevertheless, our patients do not have simple, bounded, disciplinary-specific challenges. They have challenges that are complex, that span the limits of multiple health perspectives, and that require information and perspectives from disparate disciplines to address and solve them. Although a true industry-wide shift to IPCP is likely some time in the future, the approach advocated here is akin to thinking globally and acting locally. As we await that shift, we are aware that teams can still approach interprofessional collaboration and education with a greater degree of intentionality than they may have in the past, and we have offered some research-based recommendations from the organizational literature to assist in that journey.

REFERENCES

1. D'Amour D, Ferrada-Videla M, San Martin Rodriguez L, et al. The conceptual basis for interprofessional collaboration: core concepts and theoretical frameworks. J Interprof Care 2005;19(supl):116–31.
2. American Speech-Language-Hearing Association (ASHA). ASHA's envisioned future: 2025. Available at: http://www.asha.org/About/ASHAs-Envisioned-Future/. Accessed May 31, 2017.
3. World Health Organization (WHO) Department of Human Resources for Health. Framework for action on interprofessional education & collaborative practice. Switzerland: World Health Organization; 2010.
4. Interprofessional Education Collaborative (IPEC) Expert Panel. Core competencies for interprofessional collaborative practice: 2016 update. Washington (DC): Interprofessional Education Collaborative; 2016.
5. Ogletree B. Addressing the communication and other needs of persons with severe disabilities through engaged interprofessional teams: introduction to a clinical forum. Am J Speech Lang Pathol 2017;26(2):157–61.
6. Lavin M, Ruebling R, Block M, et al. Interdisciplinary health professional education: a historical review. Adv Health Sci Educ Theory Pract 2001;6:25–47.
7. Boon H, Verhoef M, O'Hara D, et al. From parallel practice to integrative health care: a conceptual framework. BMC Health Serv Res 2014;4(1):15.
8. Interprofessional Education Collaborative (IPEC) Expert Panel. Core competencies for interprofessional collaborative practice: report of an expert panel. Washington (DC): Interprofessional Education Collaborative; 2011.
9. American Speech-Language-Hearing Association (ASHA). Final report on interprofessional education. Available at http://www.asha.org/.uploadedFiles/Report-Ad-Hoc-Committee-on-Interprofessional-Education.pdf. Accessed May 3, 2017.
10. Sylvester L, Ogletree B, Lunnen K. Cotreatment as a vehicle for interprofessional collaborative practice: physical therapists and speech-language pathologists collaborating in the care of children with severe disabilities. Am J Speech Lang Pathol 2017;26(2):206–16.

11. Kozslowski S, Bell B. Work groups and teams in organizations. Review update. In: Schmitt N, Higghouse S, editors. Handbook of psychology: vol. 12. Industrial and organizational psychology. 2nd edition. Hoboken (NJ): Wiley; 2013. p. 412–69.

12. Guzzo R, Dickson M. Teams in organizations: recent research on performance and effectiveness. Annu Rev Psychol 1996;47:307–38.

13. Katzenbach J, Smith D. The wisdom of teams: creating the high performance organization. Boston: Harvard Business Review Press; 1993.

14. McGrath J, Arrow H, Berdahl L. The study of groups: past, present, future. Pers Soc Psychol Rev 2000;4:95–105.

15. Hackman R. Leading teams: setting the stage for great performance. Boston: Harvard Business Review Press; 2002.

16. Van de Ven A, Delbecq A, Koenig R. Determinants of coordination modes within organizations. Am Sociol Rev 1976;41:322–38.

17. Burke W. Team building. In: Reddy W, Jamison K, editors. Team building: blueprints for productivity and satisfaction. Alexandria (VA): NTL Institute for Applied Behavioral Science; 1982. p. 3–14.

18. Cannon-Bowers J, Salas E, Converse S. Shared mental models in expert team decision making. In: Castellan N, editor. Individual and group decision-making. Hillsdale (NJ): Lawrence Erlbaum Associates; 1993. p. 221–46.

19. Mathieu J, Heffner T, Goodwin G, et al. Scaling the quality of teammates' mental models: equifinality and normative comparisons. J Organ Behav 2005;26: 37–56.

20. Collins J, Porras J. Organizational vision and visionary organizations. Calif Manag Rev 1991;34:30–52.

21. Dyer G, Dyer J, Dyer W. Team building: proven strategies for improving team performance. 5th edition. San Francisco (CA): Jossey-Bass; 2013.

22. Klein C, DiazGranados D, Salas E, et al. Does team building work? Small Group Research 2009;40:181–222.

23. Salas E, Rozell D, Mullen B, et al. The effect of team building on performance. Small Group Research 1999;30:309–29.

24. Mannix E, Neale M. What differences make a difference: the promise and reality of diverse teams in organizations. Psychol Sci Public Interest 2005;6: 31–55.

25. Watson W, Kumar K, Michaelson L. Cultural diversity's impact on interaction process and performance: comparing homogenous and diverse task groups. Acad Manage J 1993;36:590–602.

26. Hackman J, Oldham G. Work redesign. Reading (MA): Addison-Wesley; 1980.

27. Krantz J, Maltz M. A framework for consulting to organizational role. Consult Psychol J Pract Res 1997;49:137–51.

28. Mumford T, Van Iddekinge C, Morganson F, et al. The team role test: development and validation of a team role knowledge situational judgment test. J Appl Psychol 2008;93:250–67.

29. Beckhard R. Optimizing team-building efforts. Journal of Contemporary Business 1972;1:23–32.

30. Burke W, Noumair D. Organization development: a process of learning and changing. 3rd edition. New York: Pearson; 2015.

31. Raue S, Tang S, Weiland C, et al. The GRPI model: an approach for team development. The Systemic Excellence Group Website. Published February 18, 2013. Available at: http://www.segroup.de/library/public/Paper_Raue_Tang_Weiland_ Wenzlik_The_GRPI_Model.pdf. Accessed May 30, 2017.

32. Beckhard R, Harris R. Organizational transitions: managing complex change. Reading (MA): Addison-Wesley; 1977.
33. Marshak R. Covert processes: managing the five hidden dimensions of organization change. San Francisco (CA): Berrett-Koehler; 2006.
34. Darling M, Parry C, Moore J. Learning in the thick of it. Harv Bus Rev 2005;83(7): 84–92.
35. Cannon-Bowers J, Salas E. Team performance and training in complex environments. Curr Dir Psychol Sci 1998;7:83–7.
36. Smith-Jentsch K, Zeisig K, Acton B, et al. Team dimensional training. In: Cannon-Bowers J, Salas E, editors. Making decisions under stress: implications for individual and team training. Washington, DC: American Psychological Association; 1998. p. 271–98.
37. Schein E. Process consultation revisited: building the helping relationship. Reading (MA): Addison-Wesley; 1999.

Late Talkers

Why the Wait-and-See Approach Is Outdated

Nina Capone Singleton, PhD, CCC-SLP

KEYWORDS

- Late talkers • Wait-and-see • Early intervention • Toddlers • Language disorder
- Specific language impairment • Parent-implemented intervention • Late bloomers

KEY POINTS

- A wait-and-see approach delays referral of a child for further developmental evaluation when s/he fails a language screening in toddlerhood.
- The view that most late talkers "catch up" seems to be outdated because they do not necessarily meet their same-age peers in all aspects of development.
- Late talking can also impact early socialization and school readiness, and can place some late talkers at risk for life-long disability.
- Interprofessional education and practice supports early referral for late talkers who are at-risk.
- Advances in the science of brain development, language development and disorders, and epigenetics support early identification and intervention, not a wait-and-see approach for late talkers.

INTRODUCTION

A wait-and-see approach with late talking toddlers—that is, not referring a late talker (LT) who fails a language screening for evaluation—can occur for a number of reasons. For example, a lack of knowledge in bilingual development has led nurses to delay referrals.[1,2] Nurses have reported lack of training in screening procedures as well as in bilingual development as primary problems in following through on referring LTs for further evaluation. **Box 1** reports related issues and suggestions for serving bilingual toddlers. From a speech-language pathologist's perspective, there is a gap between what is known about LTs and their outcomes when deciding on referral of a child for

There are no commercial or financial conflicts of interests to the work. A portion of this work was supported by an American Speech-Language-Hearing Association (ASHA) Research Mentoring-Pair Travel Award granted to the author.

Department of Speech-Language Pathology, School of Health and Medical Sciences, Seton Hall University, 400 South Orange Avenue, South Orange, NJ 07079, USA

E-mail address: nina.capone@shu.edu

Pediatr Clin N Am 65 (2018) 13–29
https://doi.org/10.1016/j.pcl.2017.08.018
0031-3955/18/© 2017 Elsevier Inc. All rights reserved.

Box 1
The unique circumstance of screening bilingual children

Bilingualism raises unique challenges for professionals without interprofessional practice training to screen children under 3 years of age for potential language delay.[1,2] Challenges include:
- The linguistic variations between the child's languages themselves
- The variations of timing each language introduction
- Cultural mismatch between screener or evaluators and the child/family

Professionals may feel underprepared in the knowledge of bilingual development and in the skill of screening procedures. Lack of training can result in:
- Using the screener's primary language rather than the child's language as the screening language
- Altering the screening procedure
- A misconception that bilingual children need more time to learn 2 languages

The consequences of these actions are:
- Invalidation of screening results,
- Delay to refer the child for further evaluation, or
- To overrepresent children of individual cultural backgrounds in evaluation/treatment

The American Speech-Language-Hearing Association's position when differentiating between LANGUAGE DISORDER and a language difference[3]:
- Communication disorders will be evident in all languages used by an individual
- Account for the process of (dual) language development, proficiency, and dominance
- Fluctuation

In addition to parents, consider working alongside other caregivers, siblings, or cousins who are familiar with the child, and his or her culture and language. Discuss the processes of screening/referral for evaluation within the family's cultural framework. In some cultures, an individual's development may not take precedence over behaviors that contribute to the family unit.

Concepts to understand:
- Simultaneous bilingual—before 3 years of age, the child acquires 2 languages at the same time
- Sequential bilingual—before 3 years of age, the child learns a primary language, and after 3 years of age, the child learns a second language
- Proficiency—the degree to which the child can speak and/or comprehend with native-like competence
- Code switching— the child changes languages between phrases or sentences that is considered typical in bilingual development

---

further evaluation. The American Speech-Language-Hearing Association (ASHA) has implemented a 10-year plan to advance interprofessional education and interprofessional education practice (IPP) as part of its *Strategic Pathway to Excellence* (http://www.asha.org/uploadedFiles/ASHA-Strategic-Pathway-to-Excellence.pdf).

The aim here is to bridge some of the interprofessional education and IPP gap with what is known about LTs and their long-term outcomes so that alternatives to the wait-and-see approach will be considered. One alternative to the wait-and-see approach is to refer an LT to a state's early intervention program. IPP is well-established in the early intervention system under Part C of the Individuals with Disabilities Education Act[4] (**Box 2**). Over the short or long-term, at least 2 professionals will collaborate in service of a LT, at any given time. The following professions may be involved in managing the child's health care, overall development, and education:

- Audiology
- Medicine (eg, pediatrician, pediatric otolaryngologist)

Box 2
Part C of the Individual with Disabilities Education Act (IDEA)

Under the IDEA, the program Child Find for Infants and Toddlers seeks out children who would benefit from early intervention. Child Find is governed by early intervention regulations consistent with Part C of IDEA. Congress encourages states to participate in Part C to provide early intervention services, but it is voluntary. At this time, the 50 United States participate in programming, as do Puerto Rico and the District of Columbia. By and large, once a child is referred to a state's early intervention system by a pediatrician or caregiver, for instance, and a parent or legal guardian consents to the evaluation, an evaluation is completed (1) within a specified period of time, and (2) at least 2 evaluators must be able to assess 5 areas of development (motor, cognition, social/emotional, communication, and adaptive functioning). The established infrastructure of each state's early intervention system facilitates swift evaluation and, if eligible, the development of a plan, and interprofessional coordination of service.

Data from Individuals with Disabilities Education Improvement Act of 2004 (IDEA), Pub. L. No. 108–446, 118 Stat. 2647 (2004).

- Nursing (medical practice, school practice)
- Occupational therapy
- Physical therapy
- Psychology
- Speech-language pathology (with expertise in early intervention, school-based, private practice)
- Teaching (eg, preschool teacher, reading specialist, elementary education)

SCREENING IN THE PEDIATRICIAN'S OFFICE

The early screening of language development in the pediatrician's office serves an important public health function.[5] Early language screening is often the conduit to diagnosing primary disabilities such as autism or hearing impairment. However, early screening also identifies language delay as a primary diagnosis in its own right.[6] Fewer than 50 words at 24 months of age, for example, can be a valid reflection of language delay and general neurodevelopmental problems[6(p226)]. In their medical practice, Buschmann and colleagues[6] identified 100 late talking children between the ages of 21 and 24 months. Interprofessional evaluation in their medical office assessed health, receptive and expressive language, nonverbal cognition, and hearing. Despite comparable weight, height, and head circumference to their typical peers, the late-talking children:

- Presented with more middle ear ventilation disorders
- Reported more family histories of language disorders

Late talking children fell into 4 groups:

- Expressive language delay only (n = 61)
- Mixed receptive and expressive language delay (n = 17)
- Language delay with cognitive impairment (n = 18)
- Autism (n = 4)

The 4 subgroups of children with language delay were comparable in socioeconomic status (SES), family history of language disorders, and hearing health.

A diagnosis of autism can be a presumptive diagnosis for treatment eligibility in a state's early intervention program. However, enrollment of a child with language delay as an isolated condition can be debated. Decisions depend on percent delay or standard deviation scores on formal testing, as well as other developmental domains affected. This paper concerns this latter group of children, customarily referred to as LTs.

DEFINING THE LATE TALKER

LTs are defined by an early language delay despite typical cognition, normal sensory and motor systems, and the absence of genetic or neurologic disease.[7,8] LTs in the 18- to 35-month age range have a prevalence of approximately 15%, but late talking is not a diagnostic category.[9,10] **Box 3** defines the language delay of LTs as primarily a late emergence of vocabulary growth.

A sluggish start to vocabulary acquisition is more likely to be transient if it occurs in isolation and is identified before 18 months of age.[5,13] In contrast, toddlers are more likely to persist in language delay the older they are when identified.[12,14] At 24 months of age, 50% to 70% of toddlers could "catch up" to peers.[15,16] Miniscalco and colleagues[12] (2005) reported that 82% of toddlers who failed screenings at 30 months of age were not recovering by age 6. Indeed, screening for language delay has become the standard between the ages of 24 and 30 months of age.

LATE TALKERS CAN BECOME CHILDREN WITH LANGUAGE DISORDER OR LATE BLOOMERS

Not all LTs eventually meet their same-age peers in language performance. Some LTs persist in their language delay and receive a diagnosis of a Language Disorder in elementary school. Language disorder is a diagnostic category in the *Diagnostic and Statistical Manual of Mental Disorders*, 5th edition (DSM-V).[9] It refers to children who have difficulty acquiring and using language that is not attributed to sensory, motor, genetic, cognitive, or other factors. Diagnosing a child with Language Disorder before the age of 4 years may be difficult according to the DSM-V owing to normal variations in language development.[9,17(p43)] For example, a boy's expressive vocabulary can vary from 79 words to 511 words at 24 months of age[11] and be considered within normal limits. Children with a diagnosis of Language Disorder are also referred to in the scientific literature as having a Specific Language Impairment[8] (SLI).

Late bloomers are LTs who do converge on average language performance, according to formal tests of language, as they approach school-age. However, late bloomers perform significantly below their same-age peers without a history of late talking.[18,19]

Box 3
Vocabulary delay in late talkers

Late talker
    Thresholds of vocabulary size:
    • Sum of fewer than 50 words at 24 months of age, or
    • A vocabulary survey that falls under the 10th percentile at any age on the MacArthur-Bates Communicative Developmental Inventory: Words and Sentences form,[11] or
    • Under the 15th percentile on the Language Development Survey at any age[7];

Or
    No word combinations by 24 months of age:
    Additional screening criteria[12]:
        Poor verbal comprehension,
        Or
        Parental concern.

WHY WAIT AND SEE?

The wait-and-see approach has been subject to debate.[6,12,20–22] The origins of the wait-and-see approach include fear of harms in identifying children as possibly delayed.[23] Harms include extra time, increased effort, and anxiety associated with further testing of the child. However, speech-language pathologists report that caregiver stress can already be ongoing from anxiety that their child is not talking when expected, or from parents who differ in opinion on the issue.[24] The parent–child relationship is negatively affected by late talking. Mothers report stress associated with late talking.[17] Diagnostic labeling has also been suggested as a potential detriment (eg, social stigma, preschool placement). Diagnostic labeling by disability is not required by the Individuals with Disabilities Education Act. When children are assessed in early intervention systems, they are generally not diagnosed. Children are discussed in terms of eligibility status for intervention. The US Preventive Services Task Force found no studies and, therefore, had insufficient evidence to make a recommendation regarding the potential harms (or benefits) of screening, referral, or intervention for speech-language disorders in young children.[(23e.467)]

The wait-and-see approach may also hinge on the perception that late talking is largely "self-correcting"[12(p1799)] because a majority of LTs are viewed as simply late blooming. There are at least 3 problems with this thinking. First, although late bloomers seem to catch up on standardized test performance, *late bloomers present a weaker endowment for language and related abilities*. That is, late bloomers do not truly approximate their same-age peers in all aspects of development. Being low average, in and of itself, on a test may not be problematic. However, a small vocabulary as early as 24 months of age continues to account for a slice of variance in language and memory performance through adolescence.[5,18] The implication is that early language intervention could potentially bolster the child's long-term outcome. In turn, early intervention could impact other domains of development that rely on oral language for their development. The late bloomer's ability to converge on typical test performance, thus far reported in the literature, does not account for other functional participation activities, such as socialization with peers, or behavior regulation and executive readiness skills needed for school.[25] Further, "catching up" has been based on group averages, which obscures individual late bloomers who fall below average in select domains.[26]

Second, *late talking is a significant risk factor for Language Disorder.*[27] The number of children who were LTs and persist with a Language Disorder is not inconsequential nor does Language Disorder have a trivial impact on everyday functioning.[8,27,28] For instance, Language Disorder is heritable. Adults with a history of Language Disorder, who were then parents of late talking children, reported about their own childhood that[28]:

- They were not facile with language.
- They were often misinterpreted by adults as having lack of motivation.
- They were self-conscious.
- They could not advocate for themselves.

As adults, their childhood experiences continued to impact their verbal interactions with other adults as well as within parental contexts.

Children with Language Disorder are more likely than typical children to be victimized and to have lower self-esteem.[29,30] The functional impact of Language Disorder is life long and intergenerational.

Third, *unerring predictors remain elusive* in differentiating late bloomers from the child with Language Disorder, particularly from screening alone. However, some consistent predictors of risk or success (eg, caregiver variables) dovetail well with a model of early intervention that targets those factors specifically. A parent-implemented intervention[31] actively coaches caregivers. Further, this model is applied in the child's natural environment and contexts for the greatest functional impact. The remainder of this paper addresses:

- The 3 overarching problems of the wait-and-see approach
- The IPP movement to abandon the wait-and-see approach
- The parent-implemented model for early intervention

LATE BLOOMERS HAVE WEAK ENDOWMENT OF LANGUAGE ABILITY

By definition, late bloomers perform within age limits—many times within a low average performance range, on formal tests after having a slow start to vocabulary.[5] For many late bloomers, however, a weak endowment for language is observed throughout childhood. This weaker endowment for language is reflected as a gap in test performance between late bloomers and typical peers that does not narrow or close, nor does it sort out individual differences. The gap between these 2 groups spans a variety of language skills including:

- Vocabulary[32]
- Verb morphology[33,34] (verb endings)
- Syntax[33] (ie, sentence formulation)
- Reading[18]
- Narratives[35] (ie, story telling)

Late bloomers show slow maturation of neural processing. This is observed in event-related potential (ERP) responses to speech as early as 3 years of age through 5 years.[36] The late bloomer waveform is different. Although the typical child shows a higher proportion of ERP signals in the frontal neural region, late bloomers do not. By age 6 years, group differences in ERP responses disappear, but the gap between the late bloomers' and typical peers' test performance does not close.

Individual Analysis

Apart from the group, individual late bloomers do not reach near-typical performance on select subtests.[19,22,37] For example, Rescorla and colleagues followed late talking toddlers from 24 months through elementary school, until they were 17 years of age. Rescorla[18] (2009) reports on 26 of the late talking toddlers at age 17 years. At 17 years of age, the group tested within an average range on tests of grammar, vocabulary, memory, reading, and writing but poorer than their typical peers without the history of late talking. Still, individual late bloomers at age 17 performed below the normal range on individual subtests of the Woodcock-Johnson Psychoeducational Battery Tests of Achievement—Third Edition,[38] the Wechsler Memory Scale—Third Edition,[39] and the Comprehensive Assessment of Spoken Language,[40] when their typical peers did not:

- 15 of 26 LTs on the Verbal Paired Associates subtest of the Wechsler Memory Scale—Third Edition
- 17 of 26 LTs on the Logical Memory subtest of the Wechsler Memory Scale—Third Edition
- 4 of 26 LTs on the Writing Fluency subtest of the Woodcock-Johnson Psychoeducational Battery Tests of Achievement—Third Edition
- 4 of 26 LTs on the Syntax Construction subtest of the Comprehensive Assessment of Spoken Language

- 4 of 26 LTs on the Grammatical Judgment subtest of the Comprehensive Assessment of Spoken Language.

Other Domains

Social skills, executive function, and behavior regulation rely on prior language achievements.[25,35] By kindergarten, Aro and colleagues[25] (2014) found that late bloomers tested within the average range for language—albeit lower performance than their same-age peers, but late bloomers had:

- Greater executive function problems (eg, problems with multiple types of attention);
- More emotional and behavioral regulation problems (eg, arguing with others, impulsivity, motor restlessness)
- Fewer social skills (eg, poor cooperation, lack of appropriate assertiveness)

Typically, children transition to language as a vehicle for regulating themselves and others in the toddler and preschool years. LTs may be missing the language experiences during this critical time. Even LTs who seem to reach average language abilities by school-age subsequently have holes in the ensuing tools required for socialization and academic learning.[21,25]

LATE TALKING IS A RISK FACTOR FOR PERSISTENT LANGUAGE DISORDER

Late talking is a risk factor for persistent Language Disorder into the school-age years and the risk extends to reading disorder.[8,10,21,27,41,42] Reading is particularly vulnerable. Many LTs are re-enrolled in reading intervention at school-age after being discharged from prior language therapy.[27] At least 1 in 5 LTs will persist with Language Disorder into elementary school. Leonard's (2014), seminal book on Specific Language Impairment[8] used the term "risky"[(p151)] when writing about delaying intervention for LTs.

In typical development, the early phase of language growth is first focused on rapid vocabulary learning. For the LT, there is late emergence of vocabulary growth.[27,36] Once growth is initiated, the growth curve follows a typical trajectory for some early language skills,[27] but remains significantly below age expectation throughout childhood.[27,36] After 4 years of age, the child with Language Disorder transcends a small vocabulary size to include difficulty with word retrieval, grammar, figurative language, and larger linguistic units of discourse (eg, for cooperative learning, negotiation[43,44]). These are all language abilities needed for social and academic success. **Box 4** illustrates the association between early vocabulary and language development.

Grammatical impairments have become a clinical marker of Language Disorder[27]—specifically, failing to mark verb tense and agreement by elementary school.[52] The child with Language Disorder says "the dog bark," instead of "the dog barked" or "the dog barks." Hadley and Holt (2006)[53] potentially found an early indicator of this marker. Individual growth analysis of LTs with familial history of language impairment revealed a delay in emergence and slow growth of tense marking before 3 years of age in comparison with other LT peers.

Sentence formulations remain simple rather than complex in the child with Language Disorder.[54] From ages 8 to 16 years of age, there is a plateau in grammatical development that is also reflected in a poor ability to identify grammaticality of sentences. Rice[27] (2012) studied probands of LTs into adulthood. LTs who became children with Language Disorder presented with:

- A deceleration in grammatical development
- A premature ceiling in grammatical skill

Box 4
The importance of building a rich vocabulary early in development

Vocabulary to grammar

Relationships between early vocabulary and grammar are neither random nor dissociated.[45] Most typical children acquire an early object-dominant vocabulary. More object words in the early vocabulary correlates with a larger total vocabulary size, and subsequently the child meets early grammar milestones sooner than toddlers with fewer objects words.[45] The more object words in the early lexicon, the earlier the child will initiate language growth[46] (ie, have the word spurt) that late talkers fail to achieve by 24 months. The word spurt is important for the subsequent learning of verbs, and decontextualized talk.[45] The crux of learning verb vocabulary is acquiring the verb endings and complex sentence building. Rescorla and colleagues[32] found similar relationships between late talkers vocabulary and grammar even though the late talker vocabulary was small for age. The larger the small vocabulary, the more likely a word spurt was to occur.

Other skills

The endowment of a small vocabulary early in development continues to influence later academic skills.[36] Scheffner Hammer and colleagues (2016) found that being a late talker at 24 months was a strong predictor of 48-month receptive vocabulary size. Subsequently, having a low receptive vocabulary score at 48 months played a greater role than late talker status on school readiness for kindergarten. In Rescorla's cohort[18] of 26 late talking toddlers, expressive vocabulary size at 2 years of age accounted for 17% of the variance in vocabulary/grammar and verbal memory measures at 17 years of age.

Word Retrieval

The frequency with which a child encounters a word, says a word, and richer knowledge about a word, the more likely she or he will recall the word, and say that word when she or he needs to. These relationships are true of toddlers, preschoolers, and school-age children, as well as children with language disorder.[47–51] Proficient reading also requires easy retrieval of words from memory.[41] Language intervention provides both increased frequency and quality of vocabulary exposures needed to ease word retrieval.

LTs also come to literacy with uneven and weak[41] spoken language development. The timing of learning to read, as well as failing to read, both affect activation of the occipitotemporal lobes, where letter recognition occurs. Early vocabulary growth and timely speech processing development are linked to optimal language and reading performance at subsequent age intervals.[21,36,41] In work by Chen and associates (2016),[36] children with eventual Language Disorder, like the late bloomers discussed, were delayed in ERP response patterns from 3 through 5 years of age. By the age of 6 years, the ERP responses of children with Language Disorder also looked comparable to typical peers, but their language testing was below average. LTs are missing a sensitive period in early language development, when maturation of speech processing is necessary for advances in continuing language and literacy development.

On functional MRI, Preston and colleagues (2010)[21] found that, by elementary school, children with a history of late talking, when identifying a word to match a picture, showed reduced engagement of the following neural areas:

- Left superior temporal gyrus
- Left insula

- Subcortical structures including bilateral thalamus, right and left putamen–globus
- Pallidus, extending into the head of the caudate

In addition, the right superior parietal lobule activated for children with a history of late talking. Increased activation indicated greater effort in visual attention that was not seen in children with typical language development.

The prevalence of Language Disorder in school age children runs approximately 7% of age mates in the classroom.[8] For the reader's perspective, consider the current prevalence of autism, which receives far more media and policy attention[55]; prevalence is approximately 1.5% (Centers for Disease Control and Prevention [CDC], 2014). Not all children with Language Disorder at school age have been identified as an LT in toddlerhood.[8,56] The reason for lack of early identification is not yet known, but Poll and Miller (2013)[56] have suggested that, in addition to the late emergence of vocabulary, a second path to Language Disorder might be the toddler–preschooler who has timely emergence but a slowed rate of language after that.

ASCERTAINING RISK FOR LATE TALKERS GUIDES EARLY PREVENTION

Efforts in ascertaining risk factors for late talking and persisting Language Disorder have been ongoing, but no single reliable predictor has been found. **Boxes 5** and **6** list example predictors of late talking and Language Disorder, respectively. Family history and being male most consistently emerge as being associated with late talking and/or Language Disorder. The presence of a comprehension delay in conjunction with expressive delay at 24 months also tends to be associated with persistent Language Disorder. Bishop and coworkers (2012)[57] noted that heredity played a greater role in a LT exhibiting a Language Disorder. However, 2 important predictors of the LT who then persisted with Language Disorder at 4 years of age were:

- Poor comprehension at 20 months of age
- The parent's inability to repeat nonwords when the child was 20 months old

Why would a parent's nonword repetition (eg, repeat/teɪvak/which sounds like "tayvahk") predict a child's Language Disorder? All new words are nonwords before we learn them. Nonword repetition is a known indicator of the child's ability to learn new vocabulary.[66] First, this innate ability to process nonwords for repetition may be heritable. Second, parental nonword repetition may be indicative of a parent's

---

Box 5
Examples of risk and protective factors of late talker status

Males[10,58]

Family history of language delay[10,58,59]

Socioeconomic status[59]

Low birthweight[59]

Twin status[60]

Quality of parenting[59]

Time in day care[59]

Child's approach to learning[59]

Box 6
Example risk factors of persistent language disorder in late talkers

Poor receptive language/comprehension, and little to no gesture use[5,57,61]

Poor parent performance in repeating nonwords when child was 20 months old (Bishop, and colleagues,[57] 2012)

Suboptimal fetal growth[10]

Late talking in family members[10]

FOXP2-CNTNAP2 regulatory pathway[62]

Genetic risk for dyslexia[63,64]

Poor accuracy and slow speed of word recognition at 18 months of age[65]

---

own weak vocabulary store. That is, the child's vocabulary environment may be impoverished.

The influence of SES on late talking has varied from rearing at lower SES levels placing children at a disadvantage for timely talking to exerting no effect on the timeliness of talking.[10,58,59,65] Studies that show a large number of late bloomers "catch up" in language are limited in demographic to middle and upper middle class families as well as 2-parent households.[37] In many cases the SES of early studies is unknown. With a larger sample and broader demographic, Hammer and colleagues (2017)[59] found that children reared at lower SES levels were more likely to be LTs than children from higher SES levels. However, other variables mediated the effect of SES and those included:

- Birthweight
- Quality of parenting and childcare
- The child's own approach to learning (ie, specifically, attention)

These mediating variables—parenting, childcare, and approach to learning—are potentially amenable to intervention. Collisson and colleagues (2016)[58] found similar risk factors for late talking but also identified *protective* factors against late talking. Protective factors were:

- Informal play activities
- Shared book activities between infant–adult dyads

The protective activities against late talking are also integrated in early intervention programming.

WHY EARLY INTERVENTION AND THE USE OF PARENT-IMPLEMENTED INTERVENTION?

Intervention is studied for efficacy with LTs,[67] but not yet systematically as an outcome variable in recovery from late talking.[5] Anecdotally, Girolametto and colleagues (2001)[35] observed an association between participation in parent-implemented intervention and subsequent clinician-directed speech-language therapy, with a better "catch up" rate for the 21 LT–mother dyads they studied.

If an LT is determined eligible for early intervention, it places the child at an advantage. A parent-implemented intervention revolves around social interaction. In addition to a small vocabulary, LTs are described as serious, withdrawn, and less socially competent.[68,69] LTs are also more dependent on adults for both initiating and responding in conversations, even when compared with younger children who are matched for vocabulary size.[68] Desmarais and associates (2010)[70] identified deficits in social engagement abilities to be a part of the most impaired communication profiles they identified in LTs. Only the least impaired group of LTs they studied had intact social skills. In turn, parents adapt their communication style to fit the LT's social engagement presentation. Caregivers tend to become more directive instead of directed by their child's interests.

A parent-implemented intervention balances the interaction style in the caregiver–child dyad. **Box 7** lists some main components of a well-studied, parent-implemented intervention—the Hanen Parent Program.[71] In general, language intervention with LTs can be effective,[67] but a parent-implemented intervention shows greater effect sizes in expressive vocabulary growth when compared with other treatments (eg, requiring the child to imitate words). Parent-implemented intervention maximizes carryover of new skills including a new interacting style. The parent-implemented intervention model dovetails well with ASHA's policy on a family-centered[72] practice, addresses environmental risks, and maximizes protective factors against late talking. In a meta-analysis by Roberts and Kaiser (2011)[31] the Hanen Parent Program improved:

- Receptive and expressive language skills, generally
- Receptive and expressive vocabulary, specifically
- Expressive grammar, specifically
- Rate of communication

In a separate study, a parent-implemented intervention (Parent-Child Interaction Therapy[73]) was applied to school-age children with Language Disorder.[74] Improvements were observed in:

- Verbal initiations
- Sentence length
- Child-to-parent utterances

Caregivers who participate in early parent-implemented intervention for their LT can potentially continue this technique with positive response from their school-age child. Enriched social interactions with supportive caregivers[75] are epigenetic mechanisms that can be lifelong and have cross-generational effects. Epigenome refers to chemical modifications to genes that result from negative and positive experiences. A rich learning environment, if applied repeatedly, can leave a chemical "signature"[(p2)] on genes—the epigenome.[76]

Box 7
Components of the Hanen Program for Parents

Intervention
  Occurs in the child's natural environment
  Is child directed and routines based
  Follows the child's lead and interest to promote taking turns
  Occurs during social interactions and daily routines with caregivers
  Encourages caregivers to 'wait' and 'observe' the child
  Allows the child time to initiate gestural and verbal communication
  Encourages caregivers to respond to nonverbal and verbal communication
  Encourages caregivers to model language that matches the child's attention and interest
  Encourages caregivers to model an expansion of what the child said

Data from Manolson A. It takes two to talk: a parent's guide to helping children communicate. Toronto: The Hanen Center; 1992.

ABANDONING THE WAIT-AND-SEE APPROACH

The position of the American Academy of Pediatrics is that children under 3 years of age are to be referred from the pediatrician's office for further developmental and medical evaluation if a toddler fails developmental screening (available: https://www.aap.org/en-us/advocacy-and-policy/aap-health-initiatives/Screening/Pages/About-the-Initiative.aspx). The American Academy of Pediatrics implemented the Screening in Practices Initiative to foster the healthy care of children early in life. Under this initiative, children receive screening, referral and follow-up for developmental milestones (as well as maternal depression and social determinants of health). Standardized screening of developmental milestones occurs at 9, 18, and 30 months of age, as well as when a concern is expressed by a caregiver or is evident to the medical professional at well-child appointments. The Bright Futures Steering Committee modified the screening schedule by advocating for screening at 24 or 30 months owing to practical matters (ie, insurance, attendance[77]); autism-specific screening occurs at 18 and 24 months of age.[78] The CDC also implemented a campaign with similar goals:

- Learn the Signs. Act Early
- Available: https://www.cdc.gov/ncbddd/actearly/index.html

Medical and medically aligned health researchers advocate abandoning the wait-and-see approach.[6,12,22,79,80] New directions in brain and behavioral sciences,[21,36] and the availability of large population samples (eg, Early Childhood Longitudinal Study, Birth Cohort; ECLS-B[59]), endorse referral for further evaluation, but not a wait-and-see approach, when it comes to children who are late to talk (eg, American Academy of Pediatrics, ASHA, CDC). The ASHA advocated early referral through the Identify the Signs (available: www.identifythesigns.org) campaign. ASHA's position is that access to communication is fundamental to all children from birth and even those at-risk, and (in accordance with the World Health Organization[81]) advocate that interprofessional practice is the best approach to improving outcomes.

SUMMARY

Rescorla (2011)[5] has said that expressive language delay, like a fever, is common to many conditions.[(p141)] This article puts the spotlight on LTs with no concomitant diagnoses. Under an IPP umbrella, the wait-and-see approach is abandoned, and the LT is referred for further developmental evaluation. The IPP infrastructure is well-established under each state's early intervention program. Harms of referral were addressed or have no evidence. The crux of this article, however, reexamined the panoptic view that the majority of LTs "catch up" to their typically developing peers. New evidence shows that late bloomers demonstrate weaknesses that effect academic and social functioning. The child with Language Disorder may also be an outcome of late talking that should not be disregarded early on in the child's communication development. Late talking can impact early socialization, school readiness, and can place some children at risk for lifelong disability. Screening alone will not differentially diagnose late bloomers from children with Language Disorder. Referral for evaluation is supported by a number of interprofessional practice bodies and agencies. Parent-implemented intervention addresses some risks and maximizes protective factors against late talking. When considering referral for a LT, opt to refer for evaluation and potential intervention knowing that early intervention may result in long-term, positive outcomes for the child.

ACKNOWLEDGMENTS

The author would like to acknowledge Maria Emerson for assistance provided on early intervention policy and procedure.

REFERENCES

1. Nayeb L, Wallby T, Westerlund M, et al. Child healthcare nurses believe that bilingual children show slower language development, simplify screening procedures and delay referrals. Acta Paediatr 2015;104(2):198–205.
2. Wing C, Kohnert K, Pham G, et al. culturally consistent treatment for late talkers. Commun Disord Q 2007;20(1):20–7.
3. American Speech-Language-Hearing Association (ASHA) (n.d.). Bilingual Service Delivery (Practice Portal). Available at: www.asha.org/Practice-Portal/Professional-Issues/Bilingual-Service-Delivery. Accessed March, 9, 2017.
4. Individuals With Disabilities Education Improvement Act of 2004 (IDEA), Pub. L. No. 108–446, 118 Stat. 2647 (2004).
5. Rescorla L. Late talkers: do good predictors of outcome exist? Dev Disabil Res Rev 2011;17(2):141–50.
6. Buschmann A, Jooss B, Pietz J, et al. Children with developmental language delay at 24 months of age: results of a diagnostic work-up. Dev Med Child Neurol 2008;50(3):223–9.
7. Rescorla L. The language development survey: a screening tool for delayed language in toddlers. J Speech Hear Disord 1989;54(4):587–99.
8. Leonard L. Children with specific language impairment. 2nd edition. Cambridge (MA): A Bradford Book—The MIT Press; 2014.
9. American Psychiatric Association. Diagnostic and statistical manual of mental disorders. 5th edition. Arlington (VA): American Psychiatric Association; 2013.
10. Zubrick SR, Taylor CL, Rice ML, et al. Late language emergence at 24 months: and epidemiological study of prevalence, predictors, and covariates. J Speech Lang Hear Res 2007;50:1562–92.
11. Fenson L, Marchman V, Thal D, et al. MacArthur-bates communicative development inventories: words and sentences form MCDI. Baltimore (MD): Brookes; 1993.
12. Miniscalco C, Westerlund M, Lohmander A. Language skills at age 6 years in Swedish children screened for language delay at 2½ years of age. Acta Paediatr 2005;94(12):1798–806.
13. Westerlund M, Berglund E, Eriksson M. Can severely language delayed 3-year-olds be identified at 18-months? Evaluation of a screening version of the MacArthur-Bates Communicative Development Inventories. J Speech Lang Hear Res 2016;49:237–47.
14. Paul R. Understanding language delay: a response to van Kleeck, Gillam, and Davis. Am J Speech Lang Pathol 1997;6(2):40–9.
15. Dale PS, Price TS, Bishop DV, et al. Outcomes of early language delay. I. Predicting persistent and transient language difficulties at 3 and 4 years. J Speech Lang Hear Res 2003;46:544–60.
16. Paul R, Hernandez R, Taylor L, et al. Narrative development in late talkers: early school age. J Speech Lang Hear Res 1996;39:1295–303.
17. Hawa V, Spanoudis G. Toddlers with delayed expressive language: an overview of the characteristics, risk factors and language outcomes [review]. Res Dev Disabil 2014;35:400–7.

18. Rescorla L. Age 17 language and reading outcomes in late-talking toddlers: support for a dimensional perspective on language delay. J Speech Lang Hear Res 2009;52(1):16–30.
19. Rice M, Taylor C, Zubrick S. Language outcomes of 7-year-old children with or without a history of late language emergence at 24 months. J Speech Lang Hear Res 2008;51(2):394–407.
20. Paul R. Clinical implications of the natural history of slow expressive language development. 1996;5:5–21.
21. Preston J, Frost S, Pugh K, et al. Early and late talkers: school-age language, literacy and neurolinguistic differences. Brain 2010;133(8):2185–95.
22. van Kleeck A, Gillam R, Hamilton L, et al. The relationship between middle class parents' book- sharing discussion and their preschoolers' abstract language development. J Speech Lang Hear Res 1997;40:1261–72.
23. Siu A. Screening for speech and language delay and disorders in children aged 5 years or younger: US preventive services task force recommendation statement. Pediatrics 2015;136(2):474.
24. Pierson F. Bringing early intervention to her community. ASHA Leader 2014;19: 58–9.
25. Aro T, Laakso M, Määttä S, et al. Associations between toddler-age communication and kindergarten-age self-regulatory skills. J Speech Lang Hear Res 2014; 57(4):1405–17.
26. Roos EM, Ellis Weismer S. Language outcomes of late talking toddlers at preschool and beyond. Perspect Lang Learn Educ 2008;15(3):119–26.
27. Rice M. Toward epigenetic and gene regulation models of specific language impairment: looking for links among growth, genes, and impairments. J Neurodev Disord 2012;4(1):27.
28. Rice M. Children with specific language impairment and their families: a future view of nature plus nurture and new technologies for comprehensive language intervention strategies. Semin Speech Lang 2016;37(4):310–8.
29. Conti-Ramsden G, Botting N. Social difficulties and victimization in children with SLI at 11 years of age. J Speech Lang Hear Res 2004;47:145–61.
30. Jerome AC, Fujiki M, Brinton B, et al. Self-esteem in children with specific language impairment. J Speech Lang Hear Res 2004;45:700–14.
31. Roberts M, Kaiser A. The effectiveness of parent-implemented language interventions: a meta-analysis. Am J Speech Lang Pathol 2011;20:180–99.
32. Rescorla L, Mirak J, Singh L. Vocabulary growth in late talkers: lexical development from 2;0 to 3;0. J Child Lang 2000;27:293–311.
33. Weismer E. Typical talkers, late talkers, and children with specific language impairment: a language endowment spectrum?. In: Paul R, editor. Language disorders and development from a developmental perspective. Mahwah (NJ): Lawrence Erlbaum Associates; 2007. p. 83–101.
34. Rescorla L, Dahlsgaard K, Roberts J. Late-talking toddlers: MLU and IPSyn outcomes at 3;0 and 4;0. J Child Lang 2000;27:643–64.
35. Girolametto L, Wiigs M, Smyth R, et al. Children with a history of expressive language delay: outcomes at 5 years of age. Am J Speech Lang Pathol 2001;10: 358–69.
36. Chen Y, Tsao F, Liu H. Developmental changes in brain response to speech perception in late-talking children: a longitudinal MMR study. Dev Cogn Neurosci 2016;19:190–9.
37. Rescorla L. Language and reading outcomes to age 9 in late-talking toddlers. J Speech Lang Hear Res 2002;45(2):360–71.

38. Woodcock R, McGrew K, Mather N. Woodcock- Johnson psychoeducational battery tests of achievement. 3rd edition. Rolling Meadows (IL): Riverside; 2001.
39. Wechsler D. Wechsler memory scale. 3rd edition. San Antonio (TX): Pearson; 1997 (WMS-III).
40. Carrow-Woolfolk E. Comprehensive assessment of spoken language. Circle Pines (MN): American Guidance Service; 1999.
41. Buchweitz A. Language and reading development in the brain today: neuromarkers and the case for prediction. J Pediatr (Rio J) 2016;92(3):8–13.
42. Whitehurst G, Fischel J. Practitioner review: early developmental language delay: what, if anything, should the clinician do about it? J Child Psychol Psychiatry 1994;35(4):613–48.
43. Brinton B, Fujiki M, Higbee L. Participation in cooperative learning activities by children with specific language impairment. J Speech Lang Hear Res 1998; 41(5):1193–206.
44. Brinton B, Fujiki M, McKee L. The negotiation skills of children with specific language impairment. J Speech Lang Hear Res 1998;41:927–40.
45. Bates E, Bretherton I, Snyder L. From first words to grammar: individual differences and dissociable mechanisms. New York: Cambridge University Press; 1988.
46. Goldfield B, Reznick JS. Early lexical acquisition: rate, content, and vocabulary spurt. J Child Lang 1990;17:171–83.
47. Capone N, McGregor K. The effect of semantic representation on toddlers' word retrieval. J Speech Lang Hear Res 2005;48(6):1468–80.
48. Capone Singleton NC. Can semantic enrichment lead to naming in a word extension task? Am J Speech Lang Pathol 2012;21:279–92.
49. Gershkoff-Stowe L. Object naming, vocabulary growth, and the development of word retrieval abilities. J Mem Lang 2002;46:665–87.
50. McGregor K, Friedman R, Reilly R, et al. Semantic representation and naming in young children. J Speech Lang Hear Res 2002;45(2):332–46.
51. McGregor K, Newman R, Reilly R, et al. Semantic representation and naming in children with specific language impairment. J Speech Lang Hear Res 2002;45(5): 998–1014.
52. Rice ML, Wexler L, Hershberger S. Tense over time: the longitudinal course of tense acquisition in children with specific language impairment. J Speech Lang Hear Res 1998;41(6):1412–31.
53. Hadley PA, Holt JK. Individual differences in the onset of tense marking: a growth-curve analysis. J Speech Lang Hear Res 2006;49:984–1000.
54. Ebbels SH, van der Lely HKJ, Dockrell JE. Intervention for verb argument structure in children with persistent SLI: a randomized control trial. J Speech Lang Hear Res 2007;50:1330–49.
55. Bishop DVM, Clark B, Conti-Ramsden G, et al. RALLI: an internet campaign for raising awareness of language learning impairments. Child Lang Teach Ther 2012;28(3):259–62.
56. Poll GH, Miller CA. Late talking, typical talking, and weak language skills at middle childhood. Learn Individ Differ 2013;26:177–84.
57. Bishop D, Holt G, Line E, et al. Parental phonological memory contributes to prediction of outcome of late talkers from 20 months to 4 years: a longitudinal study of precursors of specific language impairment. J Neurodev Disord 2012;4(1):3.
58. Collisson B, Graham S, Preston J, et al. Risk and protective factors for late talking: an epidemiologic investigation. J Pediatr 2016;172:168–74.e1.

59. Hammer CS, Morgan P, Farkas G, et al. Late talkers: a population-based study of risk factors and school-readiness consequences. J Speech Lang Hear Res 2017; 60(3):607–26.

60. Reilly S, Wake M, Bavin EL, et al. Predicting language at 2-years of age: a prospective community study. Pediatrics 2007;120:1441–9.

61. Thal DJ, Tobias S, Morrison D. Language and gesture in late talkers: a 1-year follow-up. J Speech Lang Hear Res 1991;34:604–12.

62. Vernes SC, Newbury DF, Abrahams BS, et al. A functional genetic link between distinct developmental language disorders. N Engl J Med 2008;359(22):2337–45.

63. Lyytinen P, Eklund K, Lyytinen H. Language development and literacy skills in late- talking toddlers with and without familial risk for dyslexia. Ann Dyslexia 2005;55:166–92.

64. Lyytinen P, Poikkeus A, Laakso M, et al. Language development and symbolic play in children with and without familial risk for dyslexia. J Speech Lang Hear Res 2001;44:873–85.

65. Fernald A, Marchman V. Individual differences in lexical processing at 18 months predict vocabulary growth in typically developing and late-talking toddlers. Child Dev 2012;83(1):203–22.

66. Gathercole SE, Baddeley AD. Evaluation of the role of phonological STM in the development of vocabulary in children: a longitudinal study. J Mem Lang 1989; 28(2):200–13.

67. Cable A, Domsch C. Systematic review of the literature on the treatment of children with late language emergence. Int J Lang Commun Disord 2011;46(2): 138–54.

68. Bonifacio S, Girolametto L, Bulligan M, et al. Assertive and responsive conversational skills of Italian-speaking late talkers. Int J Lang Commun Disord 2007;42(5): 607–23.

69. Irwin JR, Carter AS, Briggs-Gowan MJ. The social-emotional development of "late- talking" toddlers. J Am Acad Child Adolesc Psychiatry 2002;41(11): 1324–32.

70. Desmarais C, Sylvestre A, Meyer F, et al. Three profiles of language abilities in Toddlers with an expressive vocabulary delay: variations on theme. J Speech Lang Hear Res 2010;53:699–709.

71. Manolson A. It takes two to talk: a parent's guide to helping children communicate. Toronto: The Hanen Center; 1992.

72. American Speech-Language-Hearing Association (ASHA). Roles and responsibilities of speech-language pathologists in early intervention: guidelines [guidelines]. 2008. Available at: www.asha.org/policy. Accessed October 17, 2017.

73. Eyberg S. Parent-child interaction therapy: integration of traditional and behavioral concerns. Child Fam Behav Ther 1988;10:33–46.

74. Allen J, Marshall C. Parent-Child Interaction Therapy (PCIT) in school-aged children with specific language impairment. Int J Lang Commun Disord 2011;46(4): 397–410.

75. National Scientific Council on the Developing Child. The timing and quality of early experiences combine to shape brain architecture: working paper no.5. 2007. Available at: http://www.developingchild.net. Accessed October 17, 2017.

76. National Scientific Council on the Developing Child. Early experiences can alter gene expression and affect long-term development: working paper no. 10. 2010. Available at: http://www.developingchild.net. Accessed October 17, 2017.

77. Council on Children with disabilities, Section on Developmental behavioral pediatrics, Bright futures steering committee, Medical home initiatives for Children

with special needs project advisory committee. Identifying infants and young children with developmental disorders in the medical home: an algorithm for developmental surveillance and screening. Pediatrics 2006;118(1):405–20.

78. Hassink S. AAP Statement on U.S. Preventive Services Task Force Draft Recommendation Statement on Autism Screening. 2015. Available at: AAP.org website. Accessed November 6, 2016.

79. Busari J, Weggelaar N. How to investigate and manage the child who is slow to speak. BMJ 2004;328(7434):272–6.

80. Lewis N. Our role in early intervention. ASHA Leader 2007;22(1):6–7.

81. World Health Organization. Framework for action on interprofessional education and collaborative practice. 2010. Available at: http://www.who.int/hrh/resources/framework_action/en. Accessed October 17, 2017.

A Pediatrician's Guide to Communication Disorders Secondary to Cleft Lip/Palate

CrossMark

Ann W. Kummer, PhD

KEYWORDS

- Cleft palate • Cleft lip • Speech disorders • Velopharyngeal insufficiency
- Hypernasality • Hyponasality • Compensatory speech • Craniofacial syndromes

KEY POINTS

- Cleft lip/palate can lead to feeding problems, aesthetic differences, hearing loss, dental abnormalities or malocclusion, airway obstruction, velopharyngeal insufficiency, and problems from other associated craniofacial anomalies.
- Communication disorders are common in children with cleft lip/palate. These can include speech-language delay, hearing loss, resonance disorders, nasal emission during speech, speech sound errors, and even dysphonia.
- If a communication disorder is suspected, the patient should be referred to a speech-language pathologist (preferably one associated with a craniofacial team) for evaluation.
- The biggest concern with cleft palate is the risk for velopharyngeal insufficiency, which can result in hypernasality, nasal emission of the airflow, and a speech sound disorder.
- Children born with CLP should be treated by an interdisciplinary cleft palate/craniofacial team for best outcomes.

▶ Video content accompanies this article at http://www.pediatric.theclinics.com.

INTRODUCTION

Anticipating the birth of a new baby is usually an exciting time of life. The expectant couple does many things to prepare for the baby including setting up a nursery, gathering baby clothes and diapers, and deciding on a name. The parents expect to have a "normal" baby, with 10 fingers, 10 toes, and an intact face.

Disclosure Statement: Royalties for the following textbook: Kummer AW. Cleft palate and craniofacial anomalies: effects on speech and resonance. 3rd edition. Clifton Park (NY): Cengage Learning; 2014. Royalties for a clinical device: Oral & Nasal Listener, Super Duper, Inc. Division of Speech-Language Pathology, Cincinnati Children's Hospital Medical Center, University of Cincinnati College of Medicine, 3333 Burnet Avenue, MLC 4011, Cincinnati, OH 45229, USA
E-mail address: Ann.kummer@cchmc.org

Pediatr Clin N Am 65 (2018) 31–46
https://doi.org/10.1016/j.pcl.2017.08.019 **pediatric.theclinics.com**

Unfortunately, not all babies are born with perfect structures. When a child is born with cleft lip/palate (CLP), it can be devastating to the new parents. What was expected to be a happy and exciting time becomes a stressful and emotional time for the parents and other family members. It may be impossible for the parents to initially see past the anomaly to really appreciate and bond with their newborn baby.[1,2]

Cleft lip, with or without cleft palate, is the fourth most common birth defect and the first most common facial birth defect. The prevalence of clefts has been estimated to be 1 in every 600 children born in the United States,[3] although one study showed the prevalence to be about 1 in 1000 for cleft lip, with or without cleft palate, and about 1 in 1500 for cleft lip and palate.[4] In addition, a large number of children born with isolated cleft palate have other associated craniofacial malformations. In fact, cleft palate is a characteristic of more than 400 recognized syndromes.[5] Considering the prevalence of clefts in the general population, pediatricians should have a general knowledge about the management of these patients.

This article describes how different types of clefts affect the child's function and, in particular, the child's communication abilities. This article also describes the evaluation process and various options for the treatment of affected speech. Because these children have many complicated needs over their entire growth period, it is important that they are referred by the pediatrician to a cleft palate/craniofacial team for the best care and best ultimate outcomes.

TYPES OF CLEFTS

Clefts of the lip and/or palate vary in the structures affected and in the severity (eg, length and width) of the cleft. Orofacial clefts can be of the primary palate (lip and alveolus), secondary palate (hard palate and soft palate), or both (**Box 1**, **Fig. 1**).

Box 1
Types of clefts

Orofacial clefts occur because of a delay in the migration of neural crest cells in the first trimester. This delay can result in a cleft of the primary palate, a cleft of the secondary palate, or a cleft of both.

Primary Palate (also called prepalate)

- Forms at 7 weeks' gestation
- Is anterior to the incisive foramen
- Includes the lip and alveolus
- Clefts can be:
  ○ Complete (thru the lip and alveolus to the incisive foramen) or incomplete (ie, lip only)
  ○ unilateral or bilateral

Secondary Palate

- Forms at 9 weeks' gestation
- Is posterior to the incisive foramen
- Includes the hard and soft palate (velum)
- Clefts can be:
  ○ Complete (including the uvula, velum, and hard palate to the incisive foramen), incomplete (ie, a portion of the velum only), or submucous (under the mucosa)
  ○ Midline only

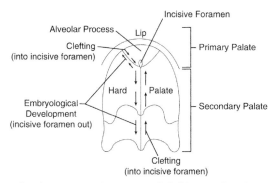

Fig. 1. Embryologic development and patterns of clefting. Embryologic development pro-ceeds from the incisive foramen out to the periphery. Clefting patterns begin at the periph-ery and follow the lines of normal embryologic fusion toward the incisive foramen to the point of that disruption. The classification of clefts as affecting either the primary palate or secondary plate is based on embryologic development, with the incisive foramen as the dividing point between the 2.

Primary palatal clefts can be unilateral (**Fig. 2**) or bilateral (**Fig. 3**), as the clefts follow the lines of the philtral ridges and the incisive suture lines. Secondary palatal clefts are midline because they follow the median palatine suture line (**Fig. 4**).

It is common to have a cleft of both the primary and secondary palate. Primary and secondary palatal clefts can be complete, in that they extend all the way to the area of the incisive foramen, or incomplete, in that they are shorter in length. Incomplete clefts of the primary palate can be as slight as a barely detectable notch in the upper lip. Incomplete clefts of the secondary palate can be as slight as a notch in the uvula, a bifid uvula, or a uvula that is hypoplastic. A submucous cleft is a case in which the oral surface of the velum is intact but there is a cleft on the nasal surface (**Fig. 5**). This cleft often affects the normal attachment of levator veli palatini muscle, which is responsible for elevating the velum during speech.

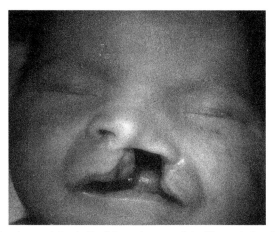

Fig. 2. Left unilateral complete cleft of the primary palate (lip and alveolus).

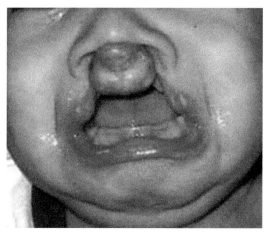

Fig. 3. Bilateral complete cleft of the primary palate (lip and alveolus). Note the prolabium (lip section that would have been the philtrum) and the isolated premaxilla bone.

EFFECTS OF CLEFTS ON COMMUNICATION AND FUNCTION

Children born with CLP are at risk for initial feeding problems, aesthetic differences, hearing loss, dental abnormalities and malocclusion, airway obstruction, velopharyngeal insufficiency, and problems caused by other associated craniofacial anomalies. These issues can lead to specific communication disorders, including the following:

- Speech-language delay
- Resonance disorders (**Box 2**)
- Nasal emission (**Box 3**)
- Speech sound (articulation) disorder
- Voice disorders (dysphonia)

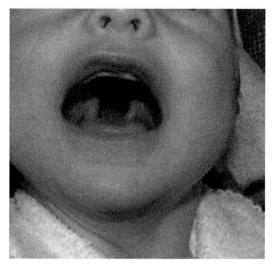

Fig. 4. Complete cleft of the secondary palate (hard palate and velum). The primary palate is unaffected.

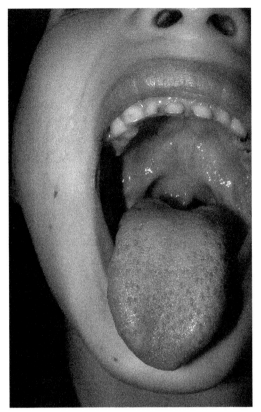

Fig. 5. Submucous cleft. Note the tenting of the velum during phonation. This is caused by abnormal insertion of the levator veli palatini muscles into the hard palate instead of into the mid portion of the velum. Note that the child is saying "aah" as in "father" and sticking his tongue out and down. This opens the back of the oral cavity for good view.

Feeding Problems

Newborns with cleft lip only rarely have difficulties with initial feeding. It is important that the nipple is placed under the bone (and not in the cleft) for compression. In contrast, newborns with cleft palate are unable to achieve suction to pull milk from the nipple.[6] As a result, breast feeding is rarely possible without supplementation. Typically, a specialized bottle is necessary in which the milk is delivered gradually to the infant without the need for suction. A consult from a feeding specialist after birth is recommended to ensure that the infant is feeding well enough to gain weight appropriately. As the child grows older, dental anomalies or malocclusion can have an effect on biting and chewing.

Aesthetic Differences

An isolated cleft lip does not directly affect function (feeding, smiling, or speech). It does impact aesthetics however. Therefore, the purpose of the lip repair (often called *cheiloplasty*) is to normalize the appearance of the upper lip. When the cleft lip extends into the nasal sill, the position, shape, and symmetry of the nose is also affected. As a

---

Box 2
Resonance disorders

Resonance is the modification of the sound generated by the vocal cords as it travels through the cavities of the vocal tract (pharyngeal cavity, oral cavity, and nasal cavity). Resonance is affected by the size and shape of the cavities. It is what provides the unique qualities to an individual's voice.

Hypernasality

- Occurs when there is too much sound resonating in the nasal cavity during speech
- Is usually caused by velopharyngeal insufficiency or an oronasal fistula
- Is most perceptible on vowels, because these sounds are voiced, relatively long in duration, and produced by altering oral resonance
- Causes voiced oral consonants to become nasalized (m/b, n/d, ng/g), which is an obligatory distortion
- Causes other consonants to be substituted by nasal sounds (ie, n/s), which is a compensatory production
- Severity depends on the size of the opening, the etiology, and even articulation

Hyponasality

- Occurs when there is not enough nasal resonance on nasal sounds (m, n, ng)
- Is caused by nasal cavity obstruction, including nasal congestion, enlarged adenoids, deviated septum, stenotic nares, choanal atresia, or maxillary retrusion that restricts pharyngeal cavity space
- Causes nasal phonemes to sound similar to their oral cognates (b/m, d/n, g/ng)

Cul-de-Sac Resonance

- Occurs when the sound resonates in a cavity (oral, pharyngeal, or nasal cavity) but cannot get out because of obstruction
- Causes the speech to sound muffled and low in volume
- There are 3 types: oral, nasal, and pharyngeal cul-de-sac resonance
  Oral Cul-de-Sac Resonance
  ○ Sound is mostly in the oral cavity
  ○ Is caused by small oral cavity size or small mouth opening (microstomia)
  ○ Parents describe speech as "mumbling" (which is not opening the mouth much)
  Nasal Cul-de-Sac Resonance
  ○ Sound is mostly in the nasal cavity
  ○ Is caused by VPI and nasal obstruction (eg, deviated septum, stenotic nares)
  ○ Is common with cleft palate and craniofacial anomalies
  Pharyngeal Cul-de-Sac Resonance
  ○ Sound is mostly in the pharynx
  ○ Is common in patients with very large tonsils, which block sound transmission to oral cavity

Mixed Nasality

- Occurs when there is hypernasality or nasal air emission on oral consonants and hyponasality on nasal consonants
- Causes include any form of nasopharyngeal obstruction (such as enlarged adenoids) and velopharyngeal insufficiency; can also be caused by childhood apraxia of speech

---

result, surgical correction of the nose is also needed. Although surgery for aesthetics may be considered cosmetic by some, it is actually important for the social and emotional needs of the patient. Our face represents who we are as individuals, and first impressions are powerful. Therefore, normalization of the facial structures is

> **Box 3**
> **Nasal emission during speech production caused by velopharyngeal insufficiency**
>
> Airflow from the lungs (with or without sound) is needed for production of pressure-sensitive consonants, such as plosives (p, b, t, d, k, g), fricatives (f, v, s, z, sh, zh, th), and affricates (ch, j). VPI causes air to leak through the velopharyngeal valve during consonant production. This can cause audible nasal emission, particularly on voiceless consonants (p, t, k, f, s, sh, ch) and affect the clarity of the speech sounds.
>
> The effect of nasal emission on speech depends on the size of the velopharyngeal (VP) opening, as noted below:
>
> - Small VP opening: Causes a loud and distracting from of nasal emission, called a nasal rustle (nasal turbulence). The sound is actually produced by bubbling of secretions as air is forced through the small opening. This increases the air pressure, which is then released with high velocity on the nasal surface of the velum. This is what causes the audible bubbling.
>
> - Large VP opening: May be barely audible or inaudible because of minimal impedance to the airflow. However, the loss of airflow through the nasal cavity causes:
>   - Low volume: Sound is absorbed in the pharynx and nasal cavity, causing the volume of speech to be reduced.
>   - Weak or omitted consonants: The greater the nasal air emission, the weaker the consonants will be because of loss of oral airflow.
>   - Short utterance length: The leak of air causes a need to increase respiratory effort and take more frequent breaths. Therefore, utterance length becomes shortened.
>   - Nasal grimace: There is a contraction seen at side of nose or at nasal bridge. This is an overflow muscle reaction to effort increase oral airflow.
>   - Compensatory articulation errors: Because of inadequate airflow in the oral cavity to produce consonants, the child may learn to produce consonants in the pharynx, where there is airflow.

medically necessary to support the patient's ability to develop normal social and communication skills.

Hearing Loss

Children with cleft palate are at increased risk for both conductive and sensorineural hearing loss. The cleft palate often causes abnormalities of the tensor veli palatini muscles, which are responsible for Eustachian tube function. Eustachian tube dysfunction can result in chronic middle ear effusion and fluctuating conductive hearing loss. Conductive hearing loss can cause a delay in speech or language development, although this delay is usually resolved quickly with treatment. Therefore, prophylactic insertion of pressure equalizing (PE) tubes is often done in patients with CLP at the time of the lip repair.

Children with associated craniofacial syndromes (ie, Treacher Collins syndrome, Stickler syndrome, 22Q 11.2 deletion syndrome [velocardiofacial syndrome]) are also at risk for anomalies of the external, middle, and inner ear. As a result, they may have a more significant conductive hearing loss or a sensorineural hearing loss, which can have a greater and more long-lasting effect on speech and language development. Constant surveillance of middle ear function and hearing, and early amplification when appropriate, is important for best outcomes for these patients.

Dental Abnormalities and Malocclusion

Children with a cleft of the primary palate that extends through the alveolus often have dental anomalies in the line of the cleft. These anomalies include supernumerary teeth or displaced teeth. Depending on the position of these teeth, they can interfere with tongue tip movement during speech production or divert the airstream laterally. Both will cause distortion of the speech.

Malocclusion is an even greater concern for speech than displaced teeth because it affects the normal relationship between the tongue tip and the alveolar ridge. The relationship is important for most speech sounds (t, d, n, l, s, z, sh, zh, ch, j).

Class II malocclusion is common in patients with Pierre Robin sequence, including cleft palate only and micrognathia (**Fig. 6**). If the micrognathia is severe, it places the tongue tip under the palate, rather than the alveolar ridge, causing difficulty producing many speech sounds.

Class III malocclusion, with maxillary retrusion and an anterior cross-bite, is common in patients with cleft lip and palate (**Fig. 7**) because of the inherent deficiency in the maxilla and possible growth restriction from the palate repair. Because the tongue rests in the mandible, it is often anterior to the alveolar ridge with this type of occlusion. Therefore, class III can also cause difficulty with the production of many speech sounds.

Whenever there are structural abnormalities within the vocal tract, it can cause either obligatory distortions or compensatory errors. Obligatory speech distortions occur when the articulation placement is correct but an abnormality of the structure interferes with the direction of the airstream, resulting in a distortion of speech.[1,2] In contrast, compensatory speech errors are the result of incorrect articulatory placement in response to (or to compensate for) abnormal structure.[1,2] Both of these are common in patients with dental abnormalities or malocclusion.

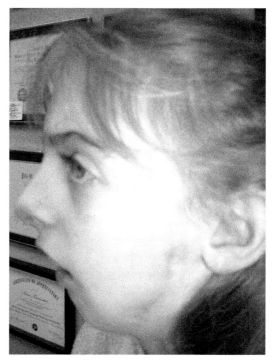

Fig. 6. Class II malocclusion caused by micrognathia associated with Pierre Robin sequence.

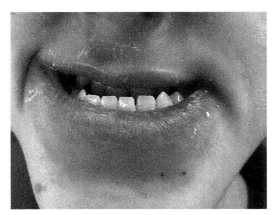

Fig. 7. Class III malocclusion with anterior crossbite caused by maxillary retrusion.

Upper Airway Obstruction

Children with cleft lip and palate are at risk for upper airway obstruction for many reasons. Those born with Pierre Robin sequence, which includes both micrognathia and glossoptosis, tend to have a very small oropharynx. This condition affects respiration but can also affect resonance. Children with unilateral cleft lip and palate often have a deviated septum, which blocks one side of the nasal cavity and can result in hyponasality. For older children and adults, the size of the nasal cavity and the depth of the pharynx may be affected by maxillary retrusion.

Patients with certain craniofacial syndromes often have both maxillary retrusion and midface deficiency, which can cause upper airway obstruction. Finally, all surgeries for velopharyngeal insufficiency partially block the nasopharynx, so there is a strong risk of upper airway obstruction and even obstructive sleep apnea postoperatively. Regardless of the cause, upper airway obstruction can cause hyponasality (Video 1) or cul-de-sac resonance.

Velopharyngeal Insufficiency

The primary purpose of the palate repair is to provide the child with an oronasal structure that supports normal speech and resonance. The palate needs to be closed to separate the nasal cavity from the oral cavity. In addition, the velopharyngeal valve, which is an important speech articulator, needs to be normalized.

The velopharyngeal valve consists of the velum (soft palate), lateral pharyngeal walls, and posterior pharyngeal wall. During nasal breathing, the velum rests against the base of the tongue (**Fig. 8**A) to allow for a patent airway. During the production of oral speech, however, it elevates and moves posteriorly to close against the pharyngeal wall (**Fig. 8**B). At the same time, the lateral pharyngeal walls move medially to close against the velum. When the velopharyngeal valve is closed, sound energy and airflow from the pharynx are directed into the oral cavity for normal oral speech.

Sound in the oral cavity is important for normal resonance and the production of vowels. In contrast, oral airflow is necessary for consonant production, particularly for pressure-sensitive phonemes, which are plosives (p, b, t, d, k, g), fricatives (f, v, s, z, sh, zh, th), and affricates (ch and j). The velopharyngeal valve closes for all oral speech sounds but opens for the 3 nasal sounds (m, n, and ng).

For normal speech, there needs to be firm and complete closure of the velopharyngeal valve during production of all oral sounds. The greatest concern for children with

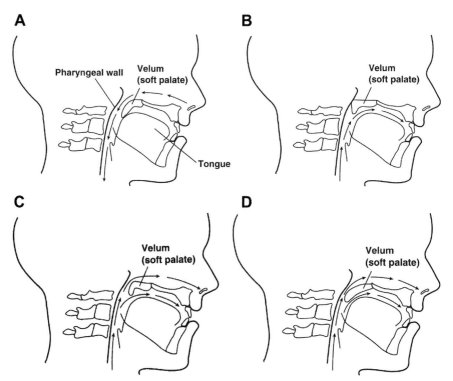

Fig. 8. (*A*) Position of the velum during normal nasal breathing. (*B*) Normal velopharyngeal closure for speech. (*C*) A short velum that causes velopharyngeal insufficiency. (*D*) Poor movement of the velum caused by a neuromuscular disorder, which cause velopharyngeal incompetence.

cleft palate is the risk for velopharyngeal insufficiency (VPI), which is defined as incomplete closure of the velopharyngeal valve caused by an abnormality of the structure (**Fig. 8**C). Unfortunately, it is estimated that 20% to 30% of children with cleft palate will still have VPI resulting in abnormal speech, despite the palatoplasty.[7]

VPI affects resonance by allowing sound to enter the nasal cavity during attempted production of oral sounds, which results in hypernasality (see **Box 2**, Video 2). VPI also results in nasal emission or the airflow during speech, which can be very audible or can affect the strength and clarity of the consonants[8] (Video 3). The effect of nasal emission on speech depends on the size of the opening (see **Box 3**).

It should be noted that, although cleft palate and submucous cleft are the most common causes of velopharyngeal dysfunction, inadequate closure of the velopharyngeal valve can also occur from other causes.[9,10] VPI can be from neurogenic causes (head trauma, stroke, or neuromuscular diseases), which cause poor movement of the velum. This type of velopharyngeal dysfunction is typically called *velopharyngeal incompetence* (also VPI) (see **Fig. 8**C). Abnormal velopharyngeal closure can even be caused by abnormal speech sound production (articulation) in the pharynx on certain speech sounds, unrelated to a structural or neuromuscular cause. Of course, differential diagnosis is critically important because velopharyngeal insufficiency/incompetence requires physical management, whereas abnormal articulation can be corrected by speech therapy alone.

Associated Craniofacial Anomalies

In contrast to isolated cleft lip or cleft lip and palate, cleft palate only is much more likely to be associated with a craniofacial syndrome that includes additional congenital anomalies.[11] As noted before, ear anomalies and hearing loss are found in several syndromes. In addition, some syndromes are associate with laryngeal anomalies, which can cause voice disorders (dysphonia). The biggest concern is that there are several syndromes with cleft palate only that have associated brain anomalies. Therefore, affected children can have developmental delays, language disorders, and cognitive disabilities.

EVALUATION
Intraoral Evaluation

An intraoral examination is important to determine if there are oral anomalies that are contributing factors to abnormal speech in patients with CLP. The examiner should evaluate the dentition and occlusion for its effect on tongue movement during speech. The position of the tongue tip relative to the alveolar ridge is particularly important. If that relationship is abnormal, there may be obligatory distortions or compensatory errors.

In addition to the anterior structures, the examiner should rule out an oronasal fistula and enlarged tonsils. If the patient has not had an overt cleft palate, the examiner should look for signs of a submucous cleft palate. Indications of a submucous cleft include a bifid or abnormal uvula, a zona pellucida (thin, bluish area in the velum), or "tenting" of the velum during phonation caused by abnormal insertion of the levator veli palatini muscle (see **Fig. 5**). It should be noted that, although an intraoral evaluation can show oral anomalies, it is not effective in evaluating velopharyngeal function because that occurs well above the oral level. Even the movement observed on the oral level does not indicate the closure of the velopharyngeal valve.

The best intraoral examination (especially with kids) is one in which a tongue blade is not used. When the examiner asks the child to say "ah," as in "father," the front of the tongue goes down, but the back of the tongue goes up. Therefore, a tongue blade is necessary to push the back of the tongue down again. A better method is to ask the child to say "aah," as in "hat," in which the back of the tongue naturally goes down. The examiner can even tell the child to try to touch his chin with his tongue, which also moves the tongue forward and out of the way[12] (see **Fig. 5**; **Fig. 9**). This technique opens the back of the mouth, giving the examiner a much better view of the tonsils, the entire velum and uvula, and the pharyngeal wall. Compliance with the examination is also improved.

Speech Screening for Pediatricians

If abnormal resonance or nasal emission are suspected during speech, there is a quick and easy screening method that can be done by the pediatrician. The examiner can use a stethoscope (without the drum) (**Fig. 10**A), a piece of suction tubing, or a bending straw (**Fig. 10**B) (which is disposable and does not need to be cleaned). One end of the tube is put in the child's nostril and then the earpiece of the stethoscope, other end of the tube, or long end of the straw is put near or in the examiner's ear.[13,14]

The following are speech samples that should be used:

To test for velopharyngeal insufficiency (hypernasality or nasal emission):

- Have the child repeat each of the following syllables as many times as possible in rapid succession: pa, ta, ka, sa.
- Have the child say the number "60" as many times as possible in rapid succession.

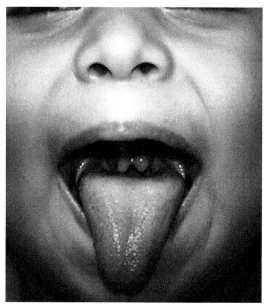

Fig. 9. This child is saying "aah" as in "father," which opens the back of the oral cavity for view. Note the bifid uvula.

If sound or airflow is heard through the tubing, this indicates an opening of the velopharyngeal valve. The child should be referred to a speech-language pathologist, preferably one associated with a craniofacial team, for a differential diagnosis and treatment recommendations.

To test for hyponasality or upper airway obstruction:
- Have the child repeat each of the following syllables as many times as possible in rapid succession: ma, na.
- Have the child say the number "90" as many times as possible in rapid succession.

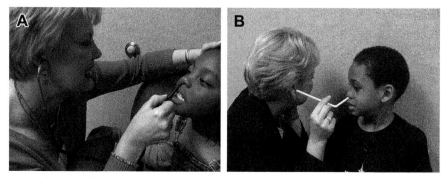

Fig. 10. (*A*) Use of a stethoscope to listen for hypernasality or nasal emission. (*B*) Use of a bending straw to listen for hypernasality or nasal emission.

If there is little to no sound coming through the tube, this indicates hyponasality and obstruction in the nasopharynx or nasal cavity. The child should be referred to an otolaryngologist for management.

Speech Pathology Evaluation

All children with a history of CLP should have an initial speech/resonance evaluation around the age of 3. This evaluation includes a perceptual assessment of speech production, resonance, and airflow on all speech sounds in various combinations.[14,15] An instrumental assessment, such as Nasometry (PENTAX Medical, Mont vale, NJ), may be done to collect objective data regarding oral versus nasal acoustic energy during the production of oral and nasal sounds. The speech pathologist will also do an intraoral examination. Finally, a nasopharyngoscopy evaluation or videofluoroscopic speech study may be recommended, based on the testing results.

Overall, the purpose of the speech/resonance evaluation is to determine the following:

- If there are placement errors owing to function or obligatory distortions and/or compensatory errors owing to abnormal structure. Obligatory distortions will self-correct with correction of the structure and therefore are not appropriate for speech therapy. Compensatory errors require speech therapy, but the therapy will not be successful until after correction of the structure.
- If the abnormality of resonance is caused by abnormal structure (ie, obstruction or VPI) or by abnormal function (such as placement of speech sounds in the pharynx, which mimics VPI), a differential diagnosis is extremely important because VPI (both kinds) requires physical management (usually surgery), whereas abnormal articulation placement requires speech therapy.

TREATMENT

The American Cleft Palate-Craniofacial Association (ACPA) strongly recommends that children with CLP should be treated by a cleft palate/craniofacial team consisting of professionals who specialize in the care of these children.[16,17] ACPA recommends that at a minimum, teams should consist of a plastic surgeon, dental professional, and speech-language pathologist. Most teams include additional professionals, including a maxillofacial surgeon, otolaryngologist, audiologist, geneticist, pulmonologist, dentist, orthodontist, psychologist or social worker, and others. Team management promotes collaborative care, best practices, and best timing of care. Even patients with noncleft VPI should be seen by a subset of these professionals for treatment.

Surgical Intervention for Velopharyngeal Insufficiency

Patients with VPI, despite the palatoplasty, require a secondary surgical procedure for correction. Several different surgical procedures can be done, including a pharyngeal flap, sphincter pharyngoplasty, Furlow Z-plasty, and pharyngeal augmentation (**Box 4**). The procedure chosen is often based on the surgeon's preference and experience.

For the best result, however, the surgical procedure for VPI should be determined based on the location of the opening and, to some extent, its size. For most patients with cleft palate and VPI, the velopharyngeal opening is in midline. Therefore, a pharyngeal flap (which closes the midline of the pharyngeal port) is usually the most effective procedure for the patient, particularly if the opening is large. If the opening is narrow or small, however, it is often best to determine the exact location of the

> **Box 4**
> **Surgical procedures to correct velopharyngeal insufficiency**
>
> The following are types of surgical procedures that can be used to correct VPI:
>
> *Pharyngeal Augmentation*
>
> • Injection of a substance (eg, fat, collagen, hydroxyapatite) in the posterior pharyngeal wall
> • Good for small, localized gaps or irregularities of the posterior pharyngeal wall
>
> *Furlow Z-Plasty*
>
> • Often used as a primary palate repair but can be used as a secondary repair to lengthen velum slightly
> • Appropriate for narrow, coronal gaps
>
> *Pharyngeal Flap*
>
> • Flap is elevated from the posterior pharyngeal wall and sutured into the velum to partially close the nasopharynx in midline. Lateral ports are left on either side for nasal breathing
> • Good for midline gaps (as in cleft palate) or deep (anterior-posterior) gaps
>
> *Sphincter Pharyngoplasty*
>
> • Posterior faucial pillars, including the palatopharyngeus muscles, are released at their base, brought posteriorly, and sutured together on the posterior pharyngeal wall to form a sphincter
> • Good for lateral gaps but closure in midline or very narrow coronal gaps

opening so that other surgical procedures can be considered (eg, a sphincter pharyngoplasty, Furlow Z-plasty, or pharyngeal injection). In these cases, viewing the opening during speech through nasopharyngoscopy is helpful in determining the procedure that has the best chance of success for the individual patient.

Prosthetic Treatment for Velopharyngeal Insufficiency

Prosthetic devices are often used in developing countries because of the lack of availability of surgery for cleft palate or VPI. In the United States, they are typically used short term or when surgery is not an option.

The most commonly used device for speech is a palatal obturator. This device looks like a dental retainer but has additional acrylic to fill a symptomatic fistula in the hard palate. If there is VPI, either a palatal lift or a speech bulb obturator can be considered. A palatal lift can be used if the velum (down to the area of the uvula) has enough length to reach the pharyngeal wall (**Fig. 11**A). The lift then holds the velum up against the posterior pharyngeal wall. If the velum is too short to reach the pharyngeal wall, a speech bulb could be used (**Fig. 11**B). The bulb of acrylic fits behind the velum and within the nasopharynx. This device is by far the hardest for the patient to use.

There are several limitations with the use of a prosthetic device for speech, including the following:

These devices:
- Require insertion and removal
- Are expensive and not always covered by insurance
- Have to be replaced periodically in children who are growing
- Can be lost or damaged
- May be uncomfortable; therefore, compliance is often poor
- Don't permanently correct the problem

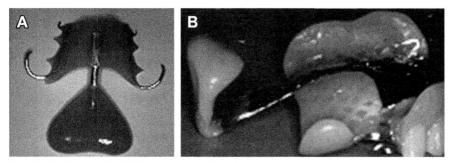

Fig. 11. (*A*) Palatal lift. (*B*) Speech bulb obturator.

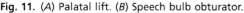

Speech Therapy for Compensatory Productions due to Velopharyngeal Insufficiency

It is important to emphasize that speech therapy cannot change abnormal structure and, therefore, cannot correct hypernasality or nasal emission caused by VPI—even if there is only a small gap! There are no exercises that are effective for treatment of VPI. Speech therapy is effective in correcting placement errors, including compensatory productions in the pharynx that cause nasal emission to persist after correction of VPI.[18] For compensatory errors, speech therapy is best done after correction of the abnormal structure that caused the development of these errors in the first place.

The success of speech treatment not only depends on the skills of the surgeon and speech-language pathologist, it also greatly depends on involvement of the family in the treatment process. Changing a speech pattern begins with motor learning. During this phase, the speech pathologist provides instructions, the child goes through a period of trial and error, and the speech pathologist provides feedback. Once the child is able to achieve the correct placement, the next step is development of motor memory. This is achieved with frequent and distributed practice sessions at home. Several short practice sessions each day will be most effective. If practice is not done at home, the progress will be slow. Motor memory is required to develop the automaticity of the speech so that the patient uses the correct speech pattern automatically, without effort or conscious thought.

SUMMARY

CLP can have a significant effect on the communication abilities of the child for a variety of reasons. Although current medical technology is not advanced enough to prevent the occurrence of CLP, most communication problems and physical anomalies associated with clefts can be improved or even corrected with the help of a professional associated with an interdisciplinary cleft palate/craniofacial team. If the patient is treated by this type of specialized team, the pediatrician will be able to reassure new parents that there is every reason for great optimism.

SUPPLEMENTARY DATA

Supplementary data related to this article can be found online at https://doi.org/10.1016/j.pcl.2017.08.019.

REFERENCES

1. Coy K, Speltz ML, Jones K. Facial appearance and attachment in infants with orofacial clefts: a replication. Cleft Palate Craniofac J 2002;39:66–72.

2. Despars J, Peter C, Borghini A, et al. Impact of a cleft lip and/or palate on maternal stress and attachment representations. Cleft Palate Craniofac J 2011; 48:419–24.

3. Cleft Palate Foundation (CPF). Genetics and you. 2008. Available at: http://cleftline.org/docs/Booklets/GEN-01.pdf. Accessed April 30, 2017.

4. International Perinatal Database of Typical Orofacial Clefts (IPDTOC) Working Group. Worldwide prevalence data on cleft lip/cleft palate. Cleft Palate Craniofac J 2011;48:66–81.

5. Gorlin R, Cohen MJ, Hennekam RCM. Syndromes of the head and neck. 4th edition. New York: Oxford University Press; 2001.

6. Miller CK. Feeding issues and interventions in infants with clefts or craniofacial syndromes. Semin Speech Lang 2011;32(2):115–26.

7. Phua YS, de Chalain T. Incidence of Oronasal Fistulae and Velopharyngeal Insufficiency After Cleft Palate Repair: An Audit of 211 Children Born Between 1990 and 2004. Cleft Palate Craniofac J 2008;45(2):172–8.

8. Kummer AW. Disorders of resonance and airflow secondary to cleft palate and/or velopharyngeal dysfunction. Semin Speech Lang 2011;32(2):141–9.

9. Kummer AW. Types and causes of velopharyngeal dysfunction. Semin Speech Lang 2011;32(2):150–8.

10. Kummer AW, Marshall J, Wilson M. Non-cleft causes of velopharyngeal dysfunction: implications for treatment. Int J Pediatr Otorhinolaryngol 2015;79(3):286–95.

11. Saal H. The genetics evaluation and common craniofacial syndromes. In: Kummer AW, editor. Cleft palate and craniofacial anomalies: effects on speech and resonance. 3rd edition. Clifton Park (NY): Cengage Learning; 2014.

12. Kummer AW. Orofacial examination. In: Kummer AW, editor. Cleft palate and craniofacial anomalies: effects on speech and resonance. 3rd edition. Clifton Park (NY): Cengage Learning; 2014.

13. Kummer AW. A screening assessment of voice, resonance, and articulation: a guide for the otolaryngologist. Curr Opin Otolaryngol Head Neck Surg 2001; 9(6):369–73.

14. Kummer AW. Perceptual assessment of resonance and velopharyngeal dysfunction. Semin Speech Lang 2011;32(2):159–67.

15. Kummer AW. Evaluation of speech and resonance for children with craniofacial anomalies. In Tatum S. & Morris L. Craniofacial surgery for the facial plastic surgeon. Facial Plast Surg Clin North Am 2016;24(4):445–51.

16. American Cleft Palate–Craniofacial Association (ACPA). Parameters for evaluation and treatment of patients with cleft lip/palate or other craniofacial anomalies. 2009. Available at: http://www.acpa-cpf.org/uploads/site/Parameters_Rev_2009.pdf. Accessed April 30, 2017.

17. American Cleft Palate–Craniofacial Association (ACPA). Standards for cleft palate and craniofacial teams. 2016. Available at: http://www.acpa-cpf.org/team_care/standards/. Accessed April 20, 2017.

18. Kummer AW. Speech therapy for errors secondary to cleft palate and velopharyngeal dysfunction. Semin Speech Lang 2011;32(2):191–9.

Supporting Children with Autism and Their Families

A Culturally Responsive Family-Driven Interprofessional Process

Marie-Christine Potvin, PhD, OTR/L[a],
Patricia A. Prelock, PhD, CCC-SLP, BCS-CL[b],*, Liliane Savard, PT, DPT, PCS[c]

KEYWORDS

- Autism spectrum disorders • Children • Interprofessional practice • Collaboration
- Coaching • Family driven • Culturally responsive • Strengths based

KEY POINTS

- Coaching in Context (CinC) is a family-driven, culturally responsive, interprofessional process that enhances functioning in everyday activities of children with autism spectrum disorder (ASD) and their families.
- Coaching can significantly increase participation in the everyday life activities of those with ASD.
- Context therapy focuses on improving a person's everyday life by changing the task demands rather than attempting to remediate the impairment of the individual.
- Goal Attainment Scaling allows the monitoring of progress toward family-driven goals and promotes family–coach collaboration in achieving these goals.
- CinC includes 3 components: connecting about the previous action plan, brainstorming potential strategies to support progress toward goals, and planning strategies to be tried.

INTRODUCTION

Children with autism spectrum disorder (ASD) may experience challenges across most International Classifications of Functioning (ICF) activities and participation domains: learning and applying knowledge, general tasks and demands (eg, following routines, handling stress, responding to demands), communication, self-care (eg, getting dressed), domestic life (eg, chores), interpersonal interactions and relationships,

[a] Philadelphia University, 4201 Henry Avenue, Philadelphia, PA 19144-5497, USA; [b] University of Vermont, Dean's Office, College of Nursing and Health Sciences, 106 Carrigan Drive, 105 Rowell Building, Burlington, VT 05405, USA; [c] University of Vermont Zippy Life Physical Therapy pllc, 32 Main Street, Suite 206, Montpelier, VT 05602, USA
* Corresponding author.
E-mail address: patricia.prelock@med.uvm.edu

Pediatr Clin N Am 65 (2018) 47–57
https://doi.org/10.1016/j.pcl.2017.08.020 **pediatric.theclinics.com**
0031-3955/18/© 2017 Elsevier Inc. All rights reserved.

major life areas (eg, school), and community life (eg, recreation and leisure).[1] Some of these challenges (eg, communication and interpersonal relationship) are core impairments of the condition and are part of the diagnostic criteria for ASD.[2] Other difficulties (eg, learning and self-care) are not part of diagnostic criteria, but are the daily life challenges resulting from the symptoms of ASD. These challenges negatively affect not only the quality of life of the child with ASD, but also that of their family.[3,4]

Numerous interventions have been designed, empirically evaluated, and clinically implemented to remediate the underlying impairments experienced by children with ASD with various degrees of success.[5] Often, however, the most important barriers to participation are not impairments, but rather the context in which an activity takes place, such as people's attitudes, the physical environment, institutional policies, and human support.[6] In fact, remediating the skills of children with ASD without consideration of contextual issues typically leads to poor skill generalization.[7] Intervention is needed that accommodates a person's impairments and modifies the environment and task demands to yield faster, greater, and more meaningful changes than intervention focused on skill remediation alone.[7–9] Intervention focused on enhancing the participation of children with ASD has the potential to increase their quality of life and that of their family.

By their nature, enhancing engagement in ICF activities and participation domains requires an interprofessional perspective, because these hinge on a child with ASD using a variety of skills that are traditionally addressed by different health professionals. For example, playing team sports requires communication, self-regulation, and social–cognitive and motor skills. Consequently, the involvement of several professions is critical to effectively address the participation needs of children with ASD and their families. Effective interprofessional practice requires collaboration from individuals of different professional backgrounds with families and their children to address their needs.[10,11]

OVERVIEW OF THE COACHING IN CONTEXT PROCESS

The Coaching in Context (CinC) process described in this article is a family-driven, culturally responsive, interprofessional process developed to enhance the functioning of children with ASD and their families in everyday activities. Family-driven practice involves families having the primary decision making role in all aspects of care including setting goals and designing, implementing, and evaluating their child's intervention plan.[12] Culturally responsive practice includes understanding a person's beliefs for the medical condition they experience, recognizing their cultural identity, developing a trusting relationship, and using strengths-based approaches.[13]

The CinC process combines 2 empirically supported interventions: coaching (a type of parent-mediated intervention) and context therapy to enhance the participation goals of those with ASD and their family. The CinC process begins with identification of family-selected participation goals and continues with family-selected and implemented strategies to realize progress toward these goals. The selected strategies prioritize modifying the task and environmental demands of an activity, rather than skill remediation. One of the interprofessional team member serves as coach to the family while collaborating with colleagues from other professions as the need arises based on a family's interest and readiness.

Coaching: Parent-Mediated Intervention

Parent-mediated intervention is a general term used to describe a variety of intervention approaches that are delivered by a parent to their child. Strong empirical evidence exists about the efficacy of parent-mediated intervention to support the development of skills, such as social emotional development, social communication, and social interactions.[14–18] In parent-mediated intervention, parents are most often provided training by a clinician so that the parent becomes the mediator of the intervention with their child; however, coaching of parents is also a parent-mediated intervention.[16]

Coaching can significantly increase participation in the everyday life activities of those with ASD.[7,19–23] With coaching, the intent is to provide supportive guidance to the family with a focus on creating an egalitarian relationship between the parent and the coach.[24] Direct instruction by the coach is minimized to encourage parents' perceptions of self-competence, and to increase their capacity to solve problems independently.[24] The coach provides emotional support and guidance to promote parent and caregiver reflection and problem solving to attain the family's and child's goals (**Box 1**).[25,26]

To be effective coaches, health professionals implementing the CinC process must be well-versed in culturally responsive practices. They must also know how to work with one another across disciplines incorporating the principles of interprofessional education and interprofessional collaborative practice. Interprofessional education assumes that different professions being educated together and learning about their respective professions from each fosters interprofessional collaborative practice and leads to improving educational and health outcomes.[11] Interprofessional collaborative practice requires different disciplines to work together to deliver the highest quality of care for children and their families within their community. An interprofessional approach is integral within the CinC process to maximize the success of children with ASD and their families in reaching their goals.

Context Therapy

The other primary component of the CinC Process is context therapy, which focuses on improving a person's everyday life by changing the parameters of a task or the environment, rather than attempting to remediate the impairment of the individual.[27] This strengths-based approach has been effective in improving the participation of children with cerebral palsy and those with ASD.[7,8] Participation in everyday activities is targeted within the context of the child's natural environment through a partnership

---

Box 1
Coaching skills

- Listen
- Empathize
- Engage
- Encourage
- Reframe
- Guide
- Be agreeable
- Be compassionate
- Be warm and friendly

Data from Graham F. Occupational performance coaching: a contemporary approach for working with parents of children with occupational challenges (Unpublished doctoral dissertation). Australia: University of Queensland; 2010 and Rush D, Shelden ML. The early childhood coaching handbook. Baltimore (MD): Paul H. Brookes Publishing Co; 2011.

between the family and the health professional.[27] However, context therapy does not determine the specific process used by health professionals when working with families. In fact, coaching should be combined with context therapy to guide this professional–parent partnership.[7] Typically, this approach has been used by occupational therapists (OTs) and physical therapists (PTs) but has relevance to speech–language pathologists (SLPs), psychologists, social workers, and other health professions likely to interface with children affected by ASD and their families.

Goal Setting

A critical aspect of, and the first step in the CinC Process is the identification of family-driven goals. These goals may be related to any domains of activity and participation that the family would like to target. It is imperative that the family selects the goals, because family goal selection increases their participation and implementation of the selected strategies.[9,28,29] The Canadian Occupational Performance Measure can be used to help families identify goals that are meaningful to them.[30] Paired with the Canadian Occupational Performance Measure, motivational interviewing techniques can also be used to help families to identify meaningful goals that are also manageable for them.[31] Motivational interviewing is a strategy used by various health professionals to promote behavioral change in a manner that is supportive and empowers the person contemplating the change. It addresses the person's feelings and thoughts, including any feelings of ambivalence, and it supports self-efficacy.[31] This strategy has been shown to be an effective family-based intervention to promote behavioral changes.[32–34] Because the achievement of family-selected activity and participation goals often requires changes in behavior, interprofessional team members using the CinC process may find motivational interviewing techniques especially useful. To illustrate each step in the CinC process, a case example is considered throughout the remainder of the article.

Case example: family-driven goals

Jamal and his family meet with an OT to whom they were referred by their pediatrician. Jamal is a 14 years old and has ASD. He lives with both of his parents and an older sibling. Jamal's pediatrician made the referral because his family expressed a desire to be able to do more family-based activities outside their home. Using coaching skills and motivational interviewing techniques, the OT engages the family in identifying their priorities for intervention using the Canadian Occupational Performance Measure. Physical activity is important to this family, who has a family membership at their local YMCA. Currently, one of Jamal's parents and his sibling, or both parents while his sibling stays at home with him, exercise at the YMCA gym a few times a week. Jamal loves to run, but is bothered by loud noises and finds it challenging to communicate with strangers. The family selected as their priority goal being able to successfully go the YMCA gym has a whole family.

A method to measure progress toward these family-selected goals should be used. Goal Attainment Scaling allows the monitoring of progress toward activity and participation goals, and promotes family–coach collaboration in achieving these goals.[35–37] Goals in Goal Attainment Scaling must meet 6 basic criteria and are rated on a 5-point progress scale (**Box 2**). Because family-selected participation goals are interprofessional in nature, successful achievement of the goals requires an interprofessional team with members who understand their respective role and responsibilities, know how to communicate across disciplines and with the family, understand the importance of a team approach to intervention, and share similar values and ethics for the delivery of care.[38]

Box 2
Creating goal attainment scaling rubrics

1. Relevant to the individual

2. Easily understandable

3. Measurable

4. Behavioral in nature

5. Attainable and realistic

6. With a specified time frame for completion

Data from McDougall J, King G. Goal attainment scaling: description, utility and applications in pediatric therapy services. 2nd edition. 2007. Available at: http://elearning.canchild.ca/dcd_pt_workshop/assets/planning-interventions-goals/goal-attainment-scaling.pdf. Accessed on April 20, 2017.

Case example: goal attainment scaling rubric

The goal selected by Jamal's family is scaled using Goal Attainment Scaling so that they can track the progress made toward their goal. Within 3 months, Jamal's family would like to be able to go to the YMCA gym as a family twice a week for 1 hour. During these outings, they would like Jamal to independently be using the gym equipment safely and appropriately for at least 50% of the time and remain quietly in the gym with a book or video game for the remainder of the time. The OT recognizes that, to support the family in reaching this goal, she will need the support of an interprofessional team that would likely include a PT, SLP, and behavioral intervention.

THE COACHING IN CONTEXT PROCESS STEP BY STEP

Once the goals are selected and scaled, the family and the coach identify the best setting in which to engage in the CinC intervention process. This process includes 3 parts: (1) connecting about what is happening in the family's life and the previous action plan, (2) brainstorming potential strategies to support progress toward the goal, and (3) making a plan of strategies that will be implemented until the next intervention session. The setting chosen is based on the family's preference and the goals themselves. It may be the family's home, neighborhood playground, the clinic, or any other location. The best location may change from week to week, depending on the family's preference and need for support.

The first intervention session begins with an initial brainstorming followed by an initial plan, because there is no previous plan. This initial session focuses on the family identifying bridges (eg, strengths to build on) and barriers to reaching a goal. In keeping with context therapy, the focus is on the environment and task demands.

Case example: initial brainstorming

Jamal's family meet with their new OT in the clinic. Jamal and his family explain that he does not like loud music and sudden noises. Jamal mostly runs on the outdoor track at school, but he has run on a treadmill in PE. The family does not know how long he can run. Jamal prefers routines and has a visual schedule at school. Jamal's father plays basketball with the assistant director of the YMCA gym. Little is known about strategies used to help with self-regulation at school. At home, Jamal spends a large amount of time in his room with headphones on playing video games. The family asked the OT to contact Jamal's school team to gather additional information that may be useful. They also suggested that the next OT visit should occur at the YMCA gym. Jamal's father offers to contact the YMCA to reserve a space to meet.

Connect

The coach and family discuss what has occurred in their life since the last intervention session and the progress made toward their goal. Assessment of progress is done through collaborative analysis of the aspects of the plan that were implemented and successful since the last session. To ensure a consistent and predictable planning process, the coach reviews the previous week's plan with the family. The coach engages the family in an explicit, rather than generalized, review of the previous plan and the aspects of the plan that the family identified as working well or those that require modification.

Case example: connect

Jamal, his family, and their OT meet for the next session at the YMCA. Jamal's family reports that they have not yet made progress toward the goal; however, they and the OT report on their progress toward the plan made during the initial brainstorming. The school PT explained that Jamal can run 5 to 7 minutes continuously before taking a break. She added that Jamal does not typically run on a treadmill at school because he tends to lose his balance while on it. The school SLP explains that Jamal reads social stories at school to help him know what is expected in specific social contexts. He offers to create one to use at the YMCA as needed. He also mentioned that Jamal was introduced to self-management strategies by his special educator. Jamal's father said that the assistant director of the YMCA was very supportive of this endeavor. Before moving on to brainstorming, the family and OT decide to walk around the YMCA gym to better understand the environment. Together they take note of the noise level, location of equipment, and other aspects of the environment and task demands that may be bridge or create barriers for Jamal to participate.

BRAINSTORM

Next, the family, with the support of their coach, brainstorm strategies that may result in progress toward the goals. Following a creative problem-solving approach,[39] the family is first encouraged to list a variety of possible ideas or strategies that may address the identified barriers in the environment or the task impacting goal achievement, while focusing on maximizing the child's intrinsic strengths. During the brainstorming phase, divergent and creative ideas are generated and recorded for all to see (ie, written on large paper or typed in a document that all participants can see). When comments about the feasibility of any proposed strategy are made, they are noted as information without dismissing the strategy. Only during the planning phase of the CinC process are these strategies analyzed for practicality, appropriateness, and likelihood of effectiveness.

Case example: brainstorm

The family wants to brainstorm possible strategies around 2 primary barriers; the noise in the gym and Jamal knowing the expected behaviors. A flip chart is used to record ideas for each barrier.

Noise	Expected Behavior at the Gym
Noise desensitization, positive behavioral support to increase tolerance of noise, noise-cancelling headphones, finding a treadmill in a quieter space within the YMCA, making the gym a quieter space.	Social stories (school SLP), comic strip conversation, self-management strategies (school special educator), if/then reward system, visual schedule.

All ideas, whether they are perceived to be realistic or not, are recorded. Resources, like the school SLP's offer to create social stories, are noted too.

Plan

During this stage, the family selects, prioritizes, and refines the strategies brainstormed during the previous step with the coach's support to create an action plan. The intent is to develop a plan that the family can implement to help the child with ASD make progress toward the goal. As in all aspects of the CinC process, this step is family driven, with the coach facilitating the process. The coach may ask the family guiding questions such as, "What strategies do you think are most likely to work?" or "What is realistic for you to try or do until our next visit?" The family is not expected to complete all the tasks in the action plan, they may ask the coach and other interprofessional team member to complete a specific task. As with all other aspects of the CinC process, the plan generation and assignment of tasks to team members is family driven.

In addition, the family may want to learn about a strategy. They may ask to be taught something specific (eg, how to do a social story), want to observe the coach implementing a strategy, or want to practice a strategy while the coach is present. Many evidence-based interventions used with those who have autism, such as comic strip conversations, may be learned most readily by a family through observation and practice. Practice of the new skills with feedback from the coach is one aspect of the professional coaching relationship.[26] If the family wants to learn about a strategy, this should be scheduled as an action step in the plan.

During this stage of the session, the family, with the support of the coach, generates a feasible action plan that is intended to foster progress toward goal attainment. The coach captures this plan in writing and provides a copy to the family.

Case example: plan

The family decides against noise desensitization and positive behavioral support to increase tolerance of noise because these strategies would take a long time before Jamal could tolerate the noise in the gym. They also decide against the noise-cancelling headphones because they are not likely to stay on Jamal's head while he is running. Finding a treadmill in a quieter space within the YMCA would defeat the purpose of having the whole family in the gym. Considering the family's relationship with the assistant director at the gym, the family decide to ask for a meeting to discuss the possibility of quiet gym hours a couple times a week during which no room-wide music would be playing and patrons would be encouraged to use the equipment quietly. The family also decides to contact the school SLP to ask him to create a social story for the gym. They will ask him what information he needs to write the social story. The family also thinks that a PT may be helpful in helping Jamal learn to use a treadmill. The OT will make a request for a PT referral and invite the PT for the next intervention session. The next session is scheduled in 1 week at the YMCA.

An interprofessional team is forming and driven by the family's self-identified action plan to achieve their own goals.

Next: Subsequent Coaching in Context Process Intervention Sessions

From this point on, each intervention session will follow the same 3 steps, connect, brainstorm, and make a plan until the family believes they have met their goal or decide to deprioritize a goal. Each session occurs in the setting that makes the most sense based on what needs to be accomplished. A variety of interprofessional team members may participate in each session depending on the strategies included in the family-selected plan. One interprofessional team member remains the coach for the family. This team member continues to use coaching skills and focus on environmental and task demands. The coach may use motivational interviewing strategies at any point in the process. In addition, the coach may use the "5 Whys" strategy (**Box 3**)

> **Box 3**
> **The "5 Whys"**
>
> 1. Write the specific challenge
> 2. Ask (and document) why the challenge might have occurred
> 3. Repeat step 2 up to 5 times to identify 5 potential causes (eg, why else?) and/or causes of the cause already identified (eg, what caused that?)
>
> *Data from* Mind Tools. Available at: https://www.mindtools.com/pages/article/newTMC_5W.htm. Accessed May 30, 2017.

to elicit reflection from the family about the potential causes of the challenges/successes and the relationship between the causes.[40] In keeping with context therapy, the coach encourages the family to consider the characteristics of the task and the environment in which the strategies were implemented in their attempt to understand the underlying causes of challenges.

> **Case example: Coaching in Context process continues**
>
> **Connect**
>
> A month has gone by. Jamal's mother meets with the OT while Jamal is using the treadmill with his father. Jamal's mother explained that the family met with a PT who assessed his endurance, balance, coordination, and treadmill skills. The PT, Jamal, and his parents agreed that Jamal would start using the treadmill at the gym for 12 minutes (ie, running for 5 minutes then 1 minute of walking, then repeat). Two, 1-hour sessions per week have been identified as trial quiet hours at the gym. The OT found that some cities have "quiet" cars in subway and trains, and "silent" dances during which attendees wear headphones with personalized music are gaining popularity. Jamal, his mother, and the school SLP wrote a social story. Jamal's mother feels that creating the social story was a great success. Jamal's mother reports that he used the treadmill during the PT assessment in the clinic, but that he has been fearful of using the treadmill in the gym earlier in the week. She also mentioned that Jamal became upset last week when the treadmill he wanted was not available.
>
> **Brainstorm**
>
> Once Jamal finishes using the gym, the steps of the CinC process continues with brainstorming related to treadmill challenges. The OT initiates the 5-Why's strategy to uncover potential reasons and solution to Jamal being able to use the treadmill with ease in the PT clinic but with difficulties at the gym. Why might this be happening? Possibilities are discussed: difference in treadmill setting (eg, inclination and speed), placement of the treadmill in the room, people walking by, different springiness to the treadmill, and so on. Possible solutions are brainstormed, too. His mother feels that, if the treadmill were oriented toward the wall, it might limit distractions but would defeat the purpose of having him socially engaged at the gym. The OT asks the family if they think that the PT should be invited to come to the gym to observe and problem solve. Jamal is visibly reluctant. His father explains that Jamal does not like having adult helpers around him. The brainstorming continues and all options are listed, even those with identified draw-backs. A dismissed option today, can become a strategy to try later.
>
> **Plan**
>
> The family decides to try a treadmill that is in a less visually stimulating part of the gym. They will make a video of Jamal using the treadmill to share with the PT for a remote consultation. The family asks the OT if they can have the next CinC session at school, so they can discuss their concern about Jamal becoming upset if the treadmill is unavailable with school personnel who have experience with this aspect of Jamal's preferences.

SUMMARY

CinC is a family-driven, culturally responsive process that is structured to facilitate family identification and achievement of their goals. The overarching intent of CinC is to provide support within a structured process that is focused on strengths to increase participation of the child with ASD and their family. The interprofessional team is key, because their collective knowledge can be used to help implement a plan that will support the coach, consider the context, and ensure success for the family and individual with ASD. Their commitment to working as a team and communicating effectively across disciplines provides support for the health professional who ultimately serves as the coach. This interprofessional approach to collaborative practice works because the disciplines share values and ethics for the delivery of the highest quality of care that is family-driven and culturally responsive.

ACKNOWLEDGMENTS

The authors thank Holly Bodony, Alex Cohen, Tammy Murray, Gillian A. Rai, Emily Slentz, Danielle Spaulding, Maura Stonberg, and Alice Symington.

REFERENCES

1. World Health Organization (WHO). International classification of functioning, disability and health: ICF. Geneva (Switzerland): World Health Organization; 2001.
2. American Psychiatric Association. Diagnostic and statistical manual of mental disorders, 5th edition (DSM-5). Washington (DC): American Psychiatric Association; 2013.
3. Potvin M-C, Snider L, Prelock PA, et al. Recreational participation of children with high functioning autism. J Autism Dev Disord 2013;43:445–57.
4. Tint A, Weiss JA. Family wellbeing of individuals with autism spectrum disorder: a scoping review. Autism 2016;20:262–75.
5. National Autism Center. National Standards Project, phase 2: addressing the need for evidence-based practice guidelines for ASD. 2015. Available at: www.nationalautismcenter.org. Accessed April 22, 2017.
6. Anaby D, Hand C, Bradley L, et al. The effect of the environment on participation: a scoping review. Disabil Rehabil 2013;35:1589–98.
7. Dunn W, Cox J, Foster L, et al. Impact of a contextual intervention on child participation and parent competence among children with autism spectrum disorders: a pretest-posttest repeated-measures design. Am J Occup Ther 2012;66:520–8.
8. Law MC, Darrah J, Pollock N, et al. Focus on function: a cluster, randomized controlled trial comparing child- versus context-focused intervention for young children with cerebral palsy. Dev Med Child Neurol 2011;53:621–9.
9. Potvin MC, Prelock PA, Snider L, et al. Promoting recreational engagement. In: Volkmar F, editor. Handbook of autism spectrum disorders. New York: Springer; 2014. p. 871–86.
10. Thistlewaite J, Nisbet G. Interprofessional education: what's the point and where we're at. Clin Teach 2007;4:67–72.
11. World Health Organization (WHO). World health statistics 2010. Geneva (Switzerland): WHO Press; 2010.
12. National Federation of Families for Children's Mental Health. Working definition of family-driven care. 2008. Available at: http://www.ffcmh.org/sites/default/files/Family%20Driven%20Care%20Definition.pdf. Accessed on April 20, 2017.

13. Mental Health in Multicultural Australia. Framework toward culturally inclusive service delivery. (n.d.). Available at: http://framework.mhima.org.au/framework/supporting-tools-and-resources/key-concepts/culturally-responsive-practice. Accessed on April 20, 2017.

14. Delaney EM, Kaiser AP. The effects of teaching parents blended communication and behavior support strategies. Behav Disord 2001;26:93–116.

15. Mahoney G, Perales F. Using relationship-focused intervention to enhance the social-emotional functioning of young children with autism spectrum disorders. Topics Early Ch Special Educ 2003;23:77–89.

16. McConachie H, Diggle T. Parent implemented early intervention for young children with autism spectrum disorder: a systematic review. J Eval Clin Pract 2007;13:120–9.

17. Moes DR, Frea WD. Contextualized behavioral support in early intervention for children with autism and their families. J Autism Dev Disord 2002;32:519–33.

18. Pickles A, LeCouteur AL, Leadbitter K, et al. Parent-mediated social communication therapy for young children with autism (PACT): long term follow-up of a randomised controlled trial. Lancet 2016. https://doi.org/10.1016/S0140-6736(16)31229-6.

19. Case-Smith J. Systematic reviews of the effectiveness of interventions used in occupational therapy early childhood services. Am J Occup Ther 2013;67:379–82.

20. Dunst C. Parent-mediated everyday child learning opportunities: I. foundations and operationalization. CASE in Point 2006;2(2):1–10.

21. Dunst CJ, Trivette MC, Hamby DW. Meta-Analysis of family centred help giving practices research. Ment Retard Dev Disabil Res Rev 2007;13:370–8.

22. Graham F, Rodger S, Ziviani J. Effectiveness of occupational performance coaching in improving children's and mothers' performance and mothers' self-competence. Am J Occup Ther 2013;61:10–8.

23. Simpson D. Coaching as a family-centred, occupational therapy intervention for autism: a literature review. J Occupational Therapy, Schools & Early Interv 2015;8(2):109–25.

24. Graham F, Rodger S, Ziviani J. Mothers' experiences of engaging in occupational performance coaching. Br J Occup Ther 2014;77:189–97.

25. Graham F. Occupational performance coaching: a contemporary approach for working with parents of children with occupational challenges [Unpublished doctoral dissertation]. Brisbane Australia: University of Queensland; 2010.

26. Rush D, Shelden ML. The early childhood coaching handbook. Baltimore (MD): Paul H. Brookes Publishing Co; 2011.

27. Darrah J, Law MC, Pollock N, et al. Context therapy: a new intervention approach for children with cerebral palsy. Dev Med Child Neurol 2011;53:615–20.

28. Østensjø S, Øien I, Fallang B. Goal-oriented rehabilitation of preschoolers with cerebral palsy—a multi-case study of combined use of the Canadian Occupational Performance Measure (COPM) and the Goal Attainment Scaling (GAS). Dev Neurorehabil 2008;11:252–9.

29. Schaaf RC, Cohn ES, Burke J, et al. Linking sensory factors to participation: establishing intervention goals with parents for children with autism spectrum disorder. Am J Occup Ther 2015;69:1–8.

30. Law M, Baptiste S, McColl M, et al. The Canadian occupational performance measure: an outcome measure for occupational therapy. Can J Occup Ther 1990;57:82–7.

31. Miller WR, Rollnick S. Motivational interviewing: helping people change. 3rd Edition. New York: The Guilford Press; 2013.
32. Broccoli S, Davoli AM, Bonvicini L, et al. Motivational interviewing to treat overweight children: 24-month follow-up of a randomized controlled trial. Pediatrics 2016;137:1–10.
33. Pakpour AH, Gellert P, Dombrowski S, et al. Motivational interviewing with parents for obesity: an RCT. Pediatrics 2015;135:e644–52.
34. Taylor RW, Cox A, Knight L, et al. A tailored family-based obesity intervention: a randomized trial. Pediatrics 2015;136:281–9.
35. Kiresuk T, Sherman R. Goal attainment scaling: a general method of evaluating comprehensive mental health programs. Community Ment Health J 1968;4: 443–53.
36. Kiresuk T, Smith A, Cardillo JE. Goal attainment scaling: applications, theory and measurement. Hillsdale (NJ): Erlbaum; 1994.
37. McDougall J, King G. Goal attainment scaling: description, utility and applications in pediatric therapy services, 2nd edition, 2007. Available at: http://elearning.canchild. ca/dcd_pt_workshop/assets/planning-interventions-goals/goal-attainment-scaling. pdf. Accessed April 20, 2017.
38. Interprofessional Education Collaborative (IPEC). Core competencies for interprofessional collaborative practice: 2016 update. Washington (DC): Interprofessional Education Collaborative; 2016.
39. Mitchell W, Kowalik T. Creative problem solving. 3rd edition. Binghamton (NY): SUNY-Binghamton Press; 1999. Available at: http://www.roe11.k12.il.us/GES% 20Stuff/Day%204/Process/Creative%20Problem%20Solving/CPS-Mitchell%20&% 20Kowalik.pdf. Accessed on April 20, 2017.
40. Zidel TG. A lean toolbox: using lean principles and techniques in healthcare. Quality Toolbox; 2006. Available at: http://services.medicine.uab.edu/publicdocuments/ anesthesiology/jc0923art1.pdf. Accessed on April 22, 2017.

Feeding Problems in Infants and Children
Assessment and Etiology

Kathleen C. Borowitz, MS, CCC-SLP[a],*, Stephen M. Borowitz, MD[b]

KEYWORDS

- Infants • Children • Feeding problems • Dysphagia • Feeding evaluation
- Development of feeding skills

KEY POINTS

- Feeding problems in infants and young children are common.
- Serious feeding problems are rare in otherwise healthy children who are growing and developing normally.
- Most serious feeding problems occur in children who have other medical, behavioral, or developmental problems.
- Serious feeding problems are best evaluated and treated by an interprofessional team of health care providers.

INTRODUCTION

Concerns about feeding problems in children have become increasingly common. It is unclear whether the incidence of feeding problems is rising or if parents and health care professionals have become more aware of them. As many as 50% of parents report their otherwise healthy children have feeding problems and as many as 80% of children with developmental delays may have difficulties feeding.[1,2] Parents worry about their child's weight gain and potential developmental consequences, get frustrated by battles during mealtime, and worry about the social impact of their children eating a limited diet. The causes and associations of feeding issues in infancy and early childhood are widely varied and almost all feeding problems are multifactorial. A feeding problem is identified when a child is not progressing through the typical course of steps to independent feeding of table foods.[3] Some children have difficulty with efficient, satisfying feeding experiences beginning at birth. Others stall or struggle

Neither author has anything to disclose.
[a] Department of Therapy Services, University of Virginia Health System, Box 386 HSC, Charlottesville, VA 22908, USA; [b] Division of Pediatric Gastroenterology, Hepatology and Nutrition, University of Virginia, Box 386 HSC, Charlottesville, VA 22908, USA
* Corresponding author.
E-mail address: kcb8t@virginia.edu

Pediatr Clin N Am 65 (2018) 59–72
https://doi.org/10.1016/j.pcl.2017.08.021
0031-3955/18/© 2017 Elsevier Inc. All rights reserved.

to move forward in accepting a variety of tastes and textures, and occasionally, children show a regression or sudden change in their feeding skills.

Despite these parental concerns, serious feeding problems that result in growth failure or nutritional deficiencies are uncommon in mostly healthy children who are developing and growing normally. In this group of children, feeding problems typically resolve with time.[4–8] A majority of these children are characterized as "picky" or "selective" eaters, meaning a child eats a limited variety of foods, is unwilling to try new foods, and/or eats slowly and deliberately.[9] Approximately half of parents characterize their preschool children as "picky eaters" and although the incidence of picky eating decreases as children get older, more than 10% of parents characterize their 6-year-old children as picky eaters.[9] Many investigators contend that picky eating in the preschool age is part of normal development and, provided the child is growing and developing normally, in a majority of cases, no interventions are warranted other than reassuring the family, scheduling regular follow-up, and reviewing basic feeding guidelines, such as maintaining a pleasant and neutral attitude throughout meals, having regular and predictable meal times, serving age-appropriate foods, encouraging self-feeding when age appropriate, and avoiding distractions during mealtimes.[7,9]

A majority of infants with more severe feeding disorders have medical and/or developmental conditions that predispose them to or are at least associated with difficulties feeding, as outlined in **Box 1**.[4–8]

Box 1
Medical conditions predisposing to infant and early childhood feeding disorders

Structural abnormalities of the aerodigestive system
- Cleft lip and/or palate (including submucosal cleft)
- Pierre Robin sequence
- Macroglossia
- Tracheoesophageal fistula
- Laryngotracheomalacia
- Laryngeal clefts
- Esophageal atresia, stricture, or stenosis
- Vascular rings/slings

Neuromuscular and developmental disorders
- Cerebral palsy
- Generalized hypotonia
  ○ Idiopathic
  ○ Due to metabolic or genetic abnormalities (eg, trisomy 21 or Prader-Willi syndrome)
- Meningomyelocele with Chiari malformations
- Congenital myopathies
- Congenital neuropathies (eg, myasthenia gravis)
- Hypoxic ischemic encephalopathy
- Metabolic encephalopathy (eg, organic academia or urea cycle defects)

Cardiorespiratory disorders
- Congenital heart disease
- Chronic lung disease/bronchopulmonary dysplasia
- Acquired vocal cord paresis

GI disorders
- Gastroesophageal reflux disease
- Food allergies
- Eosinophilic esophagitis
- Constipation
- Generalized motility disorders

Although there are several different ways to categorize the medical conditions that predispose infants and young children to having difficulties feeding, in most cases these conditions interfere with a child's ability to perform the activities of feeding as a result of

- Structural abnormalities of the face, oral cavity, or aerodigestive system
- Neuromuscular dysfunction/incoordination
- Inadequate strength and/or rapid fatigue/lack of endurance
- Inability to coordinate suck/swallow/breathe normally as a result of respiratory distress
- Nausea and/or discomfort during the feeding process

Many infants and young children with feeding disorders are diagnosed with gastro-esophageal reflux,[5] and many infants who are diagnosed with gastroesophageal reflux are reported to have feeding problems.[10–12] It seems unlikely, however, that gastro-esophageal reflux is a major causative factor of the feeding problems seen in infants and young children.[7,13] Many infants suffering from the symptoms of gastroesopha-geal reflux have symptoms of colic and constipation, and, as such, the discomfort these infants seem to experience associated with feedings may not be the result of the reflux per se but rather are the result of a more generalized motility disorder akin to visceral hyperalgesia syndrome in older children and adults. This may explain why treatment of infants with acid inhibitors does not diminish fussiness, gagging, sleep disturbance, or feeding refusal[14] and that even after the more typical symptoms of gastroesophageal reflux have resolved, many infants continue to have feeding difficulties.[11]

It is important to recognize that in healthy children, oral stimuli and feeding experi-ences early in life are pleasurable. In contrast, many children with complex medical issues may spend much of their early life in medical settings where they experience an abnormal sensory environment that often includes several aversive oral stimuli and a variety of other medical interventions that may cause a child to associate discomfort rather than pleasure with feedings. Prolonged or frequent hospitalizations as a result of premature birth, congenital cardiac defects, or gastrointestinal (GI) de-fects or disorders result in an unpredictable and abnormal sensory and social environ-ment for an infant or a young child. Conditions that require surgery, multiple diagnostic procedures, or extended periods when a child is not fed by mouth disrupt the normal progression of feeding, communication development, and social interaction. These children may have few opportunities to observe adults or other children eating and they may not experience the sights, smells, and sounds of food preparation or be able to explore foods with their hands and mouths. These simple everyday experi-ences play an important role in the sensory and social aspects of eating and they are often missed or interrupted in infants with complex or severe medical problems. These early life experiences can result in maladaptive behaviors around feeding that persist long after the painful experiences have been eliminated because once learned, abnormal motor patterns are difficult to unlearn. This may explain why the treatment of gastroesophageal reflux and the treatment of constipation are frequently not associ-ated with improvement in feeding problems.[7]

NORMAL PROGRESSION OF FEEDING SKILLS
Sucking/Drinking

At birth, term infants demonstrate root, suck, swallow, and gag reflexes that allow them to feed immediately. They are able to coordinate suck-swallow-breathe during breastfeeding or bottle-feeding, but they are dependent on caregivers for positioning. Early on, infants demonstrate a suckling pattern that is characterized by anterior-posterior movement of the tongue along with fairly wide jaw excursion. Suckling is highly automatic and reflexive. Newborns who are feeding comfortably have their arms and legs in flexion without extraneous movements, and they can maintain a quiet, alert state during breastfeeding or bottle-feeding for at least 10 minutes at a time. By 4 months of age, reflexive sucking fades, and suck-swallow becomes more voluntary. Feeding times increase to 20-25 minutes for most infants. The suckling pattern may persist until 6 months of age when more mature sucking emerges. Sucking is characterized by an up-and-down movement of the tongue and less jaw excursion. A combination of suckle and suck may be seen until 9 months of age, but children who continue to demonstrate only a suckle pattern beyond 6 months of age are not showing the typical progression. Cups are often introduced for liquid intake as early as 4 months to 6 months of age, but it is not until 11 months of age that most infants can drink from a closed cup independently and efficiently.[15,16] At between 12 months and 18 months of age, a child may still rely on biting the edge of the cup or spout to help stabilize the jaw. Most children are able to independently stabilize their jaw during cup drinking by 24 months of age and they hold the cup between their lips. Independent drinking from an open cup is usually not mastered until 18 months or 19 months of age.[15,16]

Development of Taste Preferences

Infants and young children seem to have an innate preference for sweet tasting foods that diminishes over time.[17] There is increasing evidence, however, that their taste preferences are influenced and can be modified by both in utero and postnatal exposures and experiences. In utero events and exposures seem to influence taste and flavor preferences later in life and thus modulate the intake of certain foods as a child gets older. A mother's food choices influence the flavor of the amniotic sac, and the flavors infants experience while they are in utero effect infants' flavor preferences during early infancy as well as at weaning.[18] Analogously, the foods and drinks a mother consumes while she is nursing influence the flavor of her breast milk, and these experiences effect an infants' subsequent liking and acceptance of these flavors in foods.[17,18]

There seems to be a sensitive period in infants' first several months of life during which they are receptive to a wide variety of flavors, and their taste experiences during this period influence taste preferences later in childhood.[17,19] A majority of infants less than 4 months of age are willing to drink formulas containing hydrolyzed casein, such as Pregestimil, Alimentum and Nutramigen, which are extremely bitter and have an acrid aroma; however beyond 6 months of age, infants who have never been exposed to these formulas typically refuse to drink them.[20] Infants who are fed hydrolysate formulas in the first several months of life are more willing to eat savory, sour, or bitter-tasting cereals than are infants fed standard milk-based formulas. Moreover, compared with children who were never fed a hydrolysate formula, 5-year-old children who were fed a hydrolysate formula during infancy more readily eat foods and drinks with sour or bitter tastes or aromas, such as chicken and broccoli.[17] These observations suggest infants should be exposed to a wide variety of flavors while mother is pregnant, during breast feeding, and as soon as complementary foods are added to the infant's diet.

Eating Solid Foods

Likely as a result of the slow postnatal growth and maturation, humans have developed a unique pattern of transitional feeding. Humans are the only mammals that feed their young complementary foods before weaning and are the only primates that wean offspring before they can forage independently.[21] Both the American Academy of Pediatrics and the American Academy of Family Physicians recommend that solid foods not be introduced into an infant's diet until 6 months of age.[22,23] Despite these recommendations, more than a third of mothers in the United States introduce solid foods into their infant's diet before 4 months of age and approximately 10% of mothers introduce solid foods into their infant's diet before 4 weeks of age.[24] Similarly, in a majority of nonindustrialized populations, infants are typically fed solid foods beginning between 4 months and 6 months of age, with several societies introducing solids in the first several weeks of life.[25]

Much as there seems to be a sensitive period in the first several months of life when infants readily accept varied tastes,[17,19] there also seems to be a critical or sensitive period when infants are most receptive to different food textures.[26] Children who have been exposed to lumpy or chunky solid foods before 9 months of age are more likely to eat a wide variety of fruits and vegetables and are less likely to have feeding problems at 7 years of age than are children who have not been exposed to lumpy or chunky foods until after 9 months of age. Furthermore, there is no evidence that introducing lumpy or chunky foods before 6 months of age is harmful or detrimental.[26]

Although there remains debate about when it is best to begin introducing solid foods into an infant's diet, all the available evidence suggests that provided the water and food supply are free of contamination and infants are provided adequate nutrition, there are no clear contraindications to feeding infants complementary foods at any age. Moreover, there is emerging evidence that early introduction of solid foods into infants' diet may increase their willingness to eat and variety of fruits and vegetables later in life, decrease their risk of later feeding problems,[26] and decrease their risk of developing food allergies.[27]

In most developed countries, solid foods, usually in pureed form, are typically introduced between 4 months and 6 months of age. At this age, children open their mouths for a spoon, are able to use their tongue to move the bolus of food to the back of their mouth so they can swallow it, and are able to keep food in their mouth. Oral function progresses from sucking to a phasic bite or munching, with a bite-and-release pattern at between 5 months and 6 months of age.[25] These oral skills correspond to and are dependent on the gross motor skills of good head control, sitting with support, and trunk stability. At the same time, sensory experiences to the hands and mouth increase as the fine motor skills of bringing toys to the mouth, reaching for a spoon, using palmar grasp, and transferring objects hand to hand emerge.[28] This ability to explore textures with the hands and in the mouth is likely important to a child learning to accept varying and increasing food textures.

By 7 months of age, most children can close their lips on the spoon and use their upper lip to clear the spoon. Sustained biting and the beginning of rotary chewing are usually seen between 9 months and 12 months of age and the food textures tolerated at this age progress from purees to ground or mashed table foods and some chopped table foods. By this age, most infants can sit independently. At 9 months of age, most children have a pincer grasp, which makes it easier for them to manipulate finger foods and begin self-feeding. Most babies can hold food in their hand at 8 months of age and have begun trying to use a spoon. By 15 months to 18 months, most children can feed themselves with a spoon.[15,16]

Between 8 months and 12 months, the first teeth have erupted and children can typically bite off crunchier foods. While chewing continues to mature, most children show interest and tolerance of nearly all textures without gagging. There is some evidence that chewing skills develop in response to a variety of food textures and that children who are offered more solid textures at 6 months of age have better chewing skills at 12 months of age and are more accepting of and able to adequately chew most table foods by 2 years of age.[29,30]

EVALUATING A FEEDING PROBLEM

Feeding problems in infants and young children are best evaluated by an interprofessional team. Bringing together a team of people with varied perspectives and different types of expertise provides an ability to consider influences of past and current medical problems, children's growth and development and their oral motor function, the adequacy of a child's nutritional intake, and the social milieu a child lives in. Team members can vary depending on the experience and expertise available at a particular institution. In most cases, the core team is composed of a pediatric speech-language pathologist (SLP), a pediatric occupational therapist, a registered pediatric dietician, and a pediatric gastroenterologist. The pediatric SLP evaluates oral function and a child's ability to handle an age-appropriate diet, looks for signs and symptoms of swallow dysfunction, and determines the need for and conducts an instrumental evaluation of swallow. The occupational therapist assesses fine motor development, self-feeding skills, and sensory issues. The pediatric gastroenterologist identifies, evaluates, and helps manage problems of gut motility, such as gastroesophageal reflux, poor gastric emptying, and chronic constipation as well as helping to manage enteral feeding. The registered pediatric dietician performs a comprehensive nutritional assessment, assesses the quantity and quality of dietary intake, and tries to incorporate cultural and family preferences for diet and mealtime routines. Depending on the child, additional team members could include a pediatric physical therapist, a child psychologist or psychiatrist, a pediatric social worker, a lactation consultant, and a pediatric otolaryngologist.

In a majority of cases, children should undergo a comprehensive clinical assessment of their feeding and swallowing before any more invasive assessment is performed. During this assessment, clinicians can often determine if a child's feeding problem is due to problems with the oral preparation (preparing liquid or food in the mouth to form a bolus), oral transit (moving the bolus back), or pharyngeal (initiating the swallow and moving the bolus through the pharynx) phase of swallow.[31] This information defines the need and purpose of any more invasive study, such as a videofluoroscopic swallow study (VFSS) or flexible endoscopic evaluation of swallowing (FEES). These studies are performed when there are concerns of pooling, laryngeal penetration, or aspiration. Pooling refers to the collection of secretions or residue from a food bolus that remains in the hypopharynx after a swallow. Aspiration is identified when any food material enters the airway, falling below the level of the true vocal cords. Penetration occurs when a food bolus enters the laryngeal vestibule but remains above the vocal cords.[32,33]

The first part of any feeding assessment should be performing a comprehensive history. A parent's description of the problem can reveal issues with lack of hunger signals, lengthy times to feed, frequent coughing or choking, frequent vomiting during or after meals, limited tastes and textures accepted, inability or refusal to self-feed, and crying or behavioral outbursts during meals. Strong preferences for specific foods, utensils, position during meals, or location of meals, and even who the child accepts food from suggest well-established patterns that interfere with the normal progression of acquiring feeding skills. Issues with other care routines, such as bathing, oral hygiene, and dressing, may reveal unusual or exaggerated responses to more generalized tactile input. Cultural influences about food choices and behavioral expectations need to be assessed as well.

After getting a complete understanding of a caregiver's perception of a child's current feeding difficulties, it is important to carefully review the child's growth and development, the current diet, what textures the child eats, and a description of the typical feeding environment. Current and past medical and social issues that may have effected feeding should be identified—in particular, did or does the child have any developmental disabilities or medical problems that might interfere with the normal feeding process or might predispose the child to experience pain while eating or being fed (as outlined in **Box 1**)? A history of respiratory symptoms, such as coughing or choking with feedings, chronic upper airway congestion, intermittent stridor, wheezing, or recurrent pneumonia may be the result of aspiration during eating.

As part of the assessment, a complete physical examination should also be performed. A great deal of information about a child's gross and fine motor skills, expressive and receptive language abilities, and the parents' expectations and interactive style can be gleaned by observing the child and parent while taking the history. More direct components of the physical examination should include a careful assessment of the face and oral structures, looking for facial symmetry and the shape and integrity of the hard and soft palates; movement of the velum; range of motion of the tongue, lips, and jaw; the gag reflex; and the child's ability to manage secretions. The examiner(s) should also ensure there are no unexpected abnormalities on the cardiorespiratory, abdominal and/or neurologic examinations that might predispose a child to difficulties feeding. Depending on a child's age, developmental status, and disposition/personality, it is sometimes appropriate to defer the physical examination until after a feeding observation has been conducted.

Feeding Observation

Observation of a child eating foods typically offered at home using familiar utensils provides an opportunity to assess a child's interest and response to the foods presented including the child's willingness to touch and either self-feed or accept those food in the mouth, and the oral preparation, oral and pharyngeal phases of the swallow. It is also important to try to ascertain caregivers' responses to a child during feeding. Parents may feel strong pressure to get a certain amount of food into a child when there is an early history of poor feeding and slow weight gain. Is the child allowed the opportunity to self-feed and experience new tastes and textures? Many parents find that feeding a child is more efficient than letting the child attempt self-feeding and that smoother foods fed by spoon result in faster and increased intake. On the other hand, a lack of structure and mealtime expectations can lead to a limited diet and poor intake. What is the response to a coughing or choking episode, refusal of a food, or spitting out of food? Maladaptive feeding behaviors may have been inadvertently reinforced by parental behaviors.

Assessment of Tone, Posture, and Movement

Overall muscle tone, movement patterns, and control all influence oral function. For example, head control and trunk stability are necessary to stabilize the jaw for cup drinking and to use the upper lip to clean food from a spoon. Adequate fine motor control to pick up food and bring it to the mouth or load a spoon and transfer the bite to the mouth is needed to reach certain feeding milestones. Hypertonicity or hypotonicity is often associated with exaggerated sensory responses, which may be expressed as refusal of hot or cold foods, refusal of new tastes, strong refusal or gagging with lumpy foods, thicker purees, or even soft solids. Some children show signs of seeking more intense sensation in their mouth while eating by taking large bites or overstuffing their mouths. Many of these children demonstrate clear preferences for strong tastes, such as salty or spicy foods, and/or have a preference for very crunchy textures. Lengthy chewing times, pocketing of food, or spitting out food after chewing without swallowing also suggests a sensory component to the feeding issue. Muscle tone and coordination influence the ability to manipulate liquids and solids in the mouth. A child must have the strength to bite off pieces of food; have sufficient control of the tongue to lateralize the food bolus for chewing; be able to close the lips to contain food and liquid in the mouth; and coordinate lips, tongue, jaw, and soft palate to collect the food into a bolus and propel it back for swallow.

Increases in tone and changes in movement patterns may signal pain during eating. Although it may be difficult to recognize pain with feeding in infants, extraneous movement of the arms and legs, repeated pulling off of the bottle or breast, arching or sudden fussing after only a few minutes of feeding, or lengthy comfort sucking at bottle or breast with little transfer of milk may indicate discomfort. Decreased appetite, refusal of previously accepted foods, signs of cramping, and complaint of localized pain can be associated with pain during or just after eating in children.

Vocal Quality

Assessment of vocal quality prior to observing feeding enables assessment of any changes after food or liquid has been introduced. Dysphonia—a breathy, hoarse, or raspy quality to the voice—may indicate vocal cord edema or a paralysis or weakness in one of the vocal cords. Decreased vocal cord function places a child at risk for aspiration. During eating, congested sounds at the level of the larynx, a wet or gurgling voice, throat clearing, coughing, or multiple swallows to clear one bite suggest difficulty during the pharyngeal phase of the swallow and raise concerns for pooling, penetration, or aspiration even in the absence of a history of respiratory symptoms.

Videofluoroscopic Swallow Study and Flexible Endoscopic Evaluation of Swallow

A clinical feeding evaluation may reveal signs or behaviors suggesting swallow difficulty; however, an instrumental evaluation of swallow is the only way to objectively confirm laryngeal penetration or aspiration. Instrumental assessment of swallow function can be accomplished by videofluoroscopy or by endoscopy.[32] VFSS (sometimes called a modified barium swallow) is conducted in the fluoroscopy suite with an SLP and radiologist present. As much as possible, the child is positioned in the usual feeding position. Infants are usually positioned in an infant seat in a semireclined position and older children are put into a seated position and provided with lateral or head support as needed. Food and liquid are mixed with barium and presented to the child in the usual manner. The image is lateral, with the oral cavity and neck in view. VFSS allows a dynamic view of the oral preparatory, oral, pharyngeal, and upper esophageal phases of swallow.[34]

FEES is done at the bedside or in a clinic setting by an SLP with advanced training and experience in the procedure.[35] Infants can be positioned in an infant seat or held in a typical feeding position by a parent or care provider. Older children are seated in a chair or in a parent's lap. A small flexible endoscope is inserted through the nose to allow visualization of the pharyngeal and laryngeal structures. With the scope in place, the child can be fed a typical meal. This can be breastfeeding or bottle-feeding, drinking from a cup, and/or eating solid foods.[36] The view through the scope is primarily superior, looking down into the laryngeal vestibule, thus allowing direct visualization of the nasopharynx, oropharynx, hypopharynx, and larynx during swallows. The oral and esophageal phases of the swallow cannot be seen with this technique.

There are advantages, disadvantages, and limitations to both of these assessments:

- VFSS gives specific information about the oral phase of swallow, which may be key in determining the cause of the swallowing problem. It also provides a view of the passage of the bolus through the structures during the entire swallow.
- The oral phase cannot be viewed with FEES, and there is a white-out period during the swallow when tissues contract and obscure the view of the bolus and structures.
- FEES provides information about laryngeal anatomy and function and about secretion management that VFSS does not and also allows for a longer view just before and immediately after the swallow.
- VFSS can usually be completed with children of any age whereas FEES may be limited to children under 12 months and older than 4 years because it requires a child's cooperation for the scope to be inserted. Babies can usually be quickly calmed with the presentation of the bottle, and children old enough to follow directions are often interested in the video and the camera and can often be coaxed into allowing the scope to be passed.
- Food taken during VFSS must be mixed with barium, resulting in a change in taste and texture, whereas plain food or food with dye added to improve visibility is used during FEES.
- Although FEES is invasive, it is not associated with any ionizing radiation so can be repeated multiple times without risk and can be used to view an entire feeding.
- VFSS is a less invasive procedure but does expose children to ionizing radiation so must be time-limited. Most recent information suggests the long-term effects of radiation exposure are greatest in younger children. Reported effective doses for a typical VFSS in a child vary widely ranging from 0.08 mSv to 0.8 mSv. In comparison, the dose of a typical chest radiograph is 0.05 mSv.[34,37,38] A screening time of 2 minutes to 3 minutes has been reported to be required to complete an evaluation, including a variety of food textures. Turning the fluoroscopy on and off during the study, limiting the number of swallows observed, and using a lower fluoroscopy pulse rate can limit the radiation dose. Ensuring that the study is done in a facility adhering to keeping exposure as low as reasonably achievable (ALARA), with pediatric radiologists and experienced SLPs and avoiding repeated studies, especially completed only weeks or months apart, is crucial to protecting children.

INTERVENTION

Impressions from the clinical examination and any instrumental evaluation findings direct intervention strategies. The primary goal of any intervention is to help a child achieve age-appropriate feeding skills through positive feeding experiences while ensuring swallow safety and adequate nutrition and growth. Therapy may focus on behavioral interventions, oral motor treatments, physical and sensory treatments, adjustments to diet, and the methods of intake or a combination of these approaches.

The family must collaborate with any behavioral interventions to reinforce appropriate responses to food during mealtimes and reduce interfering behaviors to be successful. Oral motor treatment to improve strength, movement, and coordination of the lips, tongue, jaw, soft palate, and pharynx may involve sensory stimulation to these areas as well as resistance, chewing, or swallowing exercises. Physical and occupational therapy may complement feeding therapy by the SLP and help a child develop postural control and self-feeding abilities and decrease aversive responses to tactile stimulation to the hands and mouth.

Modifications of the diet may include changing the viscosity of liquids, increasing or decreasing the consistency of solids offered, and adding supplemental feedings (eg, tube feedings, calorically dense formulas, or drinks) as needed. Changes during oral intake, such as altering position for feedings; altering the bottle nipple, cup, or straw to reduce or increase the flow rate; introducing compensatory maneuvers to improve bolus movement and control during swallow; and systematic introduction of new tastes and textures can be guided by the SLP or the therapy team.[39]

SOME REPRESENTATIVE CASE STUDIES
Case 1

KA is a 2-week-old boy with a hypoplastic aortic arch and slightly hypoplastic aortic valve who underwent reconstructive surgery during the first several days of life. He was extubated 4 days after surgery. The following day, the medical team consulted the SLP. During her consultation she noted a dysphonic cry and hyperactive gag; however, he was able to latch onto the bottle nipple and demonstrated short sucking bursts. His lip seal on the nipple was poor and he quickly showed signs of fatigue. He took only 5 mL by mouth during his initial feeding session but he did not cough or develop worsening congestion.

During a session 2 days later, his hyperactive gag had diminished and he latched rapidly to the nipple and had a more vigorous suck on the bottle; however, this more effective extraction of milk from the bottle was associated with periodic coughing during the feeding. His voice remained dysphonic and his cough was weak. The feeding trial was discontinued because of concerns for laryngeal penetration and/ or aspiration. The SLP recommended a pediatric otolaryngology consultation because of concerns for vocal cord paralysis or paresis associated with his cardiac surgery.

FEES was completed by the SLP with the pediatric otolaryngologist in attendance. View of the laryngeal vestibule demonstrated decreased mobility of the left vocal cord. Penetration and aspiration were observed while the child was fed thin liquid from a slow-flow nipple as well as an extra slow-flow nipple. When he was fed slightly thickened liquid from a slow-flow nipple and he was positioned in a side-lying position with his right side down to promote more medial positioning of his left vocal cord, he was better able to protect his airway and he had only episodic laryngeal penetration and no aspiration. He was discharged from the hospital a week later feeding in this manner without any clinical suspicion of laryngeal penetration or aspiration.

Case 2

SB is a 3-month-old boy who was the product of an uncomplicated term pregnancy, labor, and delivery. At a week of age he began experiencing repeated bouts of what seemed to be abdominal pain associated with eating and frequent bouts of vomiting. These symptoms worsened over time. He was initially breastfed and nursed vigorously for 5 minutes before suddenly pulling off the breast, arching, and crying. His mother eliminated a wide variety of foods from her diet without any improvement in his symptoms. He was treated with probiotics, ranitidine, and omeprazole without improvement. Pyloric ultrasound and upper GI series were normal. At 2 months of age, his mother decided to stop breastfeeding and commence bottle-feedings, hoping feedings would become less stressful for both her and her baby. His symptoms did not improve with a protein hydrolysate formula or an amino acid–based formula. The family tried different bottles and nipples without any change in his symptoms. His parents observed that he fed best and seemed most comfortable feeding when he was nearly asleep. Despite his feeding difficulties, SB continued to grow and develop.

On examination he was fussy but consolable. His weight was at the 25th percentile for age, his height at the 50th percentile, and his head circumference at the 50th percentile. His physical examination was entirely normal, including his oral examination. He had frequent episodes of crying and flailing while being held by his mother but quieted when put into a semireclined position and offered a bottle. He showed difficulty establishing a latch with frantic and disorganized movements but was able to latch and immediately showed vigorous, rhythmic sucking with a calm state for several minutes, consuming approximately 20 mL before suddenly pulling away from the bottle and arching and crying. He calmed after a minute or so and resumed feeding but his sucking bursts continued to be interspersed with crying/agitation and pulling off the nipple. His mother reported this pattern typical of a feeding at home, which often took up to an hour to complete. No vocal changes, congestion, or signs of penetration or aspiration were observed during feeding and, when actively sucking, SB was able to efficiently transfer milk from his bottle.

Based on his history, previous evaluation, and feeding assessment, there was no need for instrumental evaluation of his swallowing mechanism. His feeding difficulties seemed to be the result of GI discomfort associated with feeding. Although he had symptoms consistent with gastroesophageal reflux, it seemed unlikely this was the source of his discomfort, given numerous formula changes and treatment with acid inhibitors did not offer him relief. Rather, he seemed to be suffering from extreme colic/visceral hyperalgesia. He was treated with a low dose of gabapentin and within 5 days of starting this medication, his discomfort with feeding abated. At 6 months of age, the gabapentin was discontinued and he continued to feed well from the bottle and began eating solid foods without any difficulty or discomfort.

Case 3

JW is an 18-month-old boy without any history of serious illnesses who has been growing and developing normally. He was referred to the feeding clinic because he has been coughing and choking when he eats since he began eating table foods at 10 months of age. His coughing episodes frequently result in post-tussive vomiting. He had no problems with coughing, choking, or vomiting before solid foods were added into his diet. A chest radiograph was normal, and an upper GI series demonstrated normal esophageal anatomy and motility.

JW's parents state that he coughs at nearly every meal and that even after he has a bout of post-tussive vomiting, he resumes eating. During her feeding evaluation, immediately after JW ate a cracker, the SLP heard congestion at the level of the larynx and a wet vocal quality. During subsequent food trials, there was a suggestion of pooling and penetration as his congestion and vocal symptoms increased, and he would periodically cough. He did not seem to be in any discomfort, and he remained willing to eat. His parents had a tendency to present JW large pieces of solid foods in rapid succession.

Although there was no history of recurrent pneumonia or any other chronic or recurrent respiratory symptoms, the SLP was worried about the possibility of decreased sensation, pharyngeal swallow dysfunction, and chronic aspiration and recommended performing VFSS. She recommended performing VFSS rather than FEES because, given his age and demeanor, it was unlikely he would be able to cooperate with FEES. VFSS demonstrated poor oral control of boluses of hard solids that required chewing and this resulted in premature spillage of the bolus into the hypopharynx, delayed triggering of his swallow, and numerous episodes of penetration; however, no aspiration was seen.

Based on these findings, the authors recommended downgrading JW's diet to smooth or soft solids and offering chopped or ground higher-texture solids in small bites. JW was also referred for speech and occupational therapy services to provide him with sensory stimulation to improve his oral/pharyngeal sensory responses to higher-textured foods, develop better chewing skills and improve JW's self-feeding skills.

Case 4

AP is an 8-year-old girl who has been healthy and growing and developing normally. She had no history of asthma or other respiratory symptoms, eczema, or any problems swallowing. She was referred to the feeding clinic because of a 6-week history of refusing to eat any solid foods. Her refusal to eat solid food began immediately after she choked on a piece of steak for which her father performed the Heimlich maneuver. Since then, she had consistently refused to eat any solid foods, including purees, complaining that the food "gets stuck" in her throat. She continued to drink liquids without any choking, gagging, or coughing. As a result of her refusal to eat any solid foods, she lost 7% of her body weight. Given she was entirely normal and had no difficulties eating or swallowing prior to her choking episode, it seemed most appropriate to perform a clinical evaluation prior to any instrumental evaluation of her swallowing mechanism or her esophagus. In the clinic, she reported a sense of her "throat closing" and an inability to swallow the food. After acknowledging and validating her sense of fear of choking, the SLP explained that fear and anxiety would produce tension in the muscles of her throat, which would indeed make it hard to swallow. The SLP then led her through several breathing exercises to help her relax, and together they practiced swallowing beginning with liquids and then moving to purees, soft solids, and finally hard solids. Using the relaxation breathing she had learned, taking very small bites, chewing thoroughly, and using liquid wash after each bite, she was able to successfully swallow each consistency. Throughout the session, the SLP continuously assessed her swallow and did not see any signs of swallow dysfunction, pain, or obstruction. AP's confidence increased after she successfully swallowed each solid texture. She was given specific instructions for home oral intake using the techniques she had learned and practiced in clinic. Her mother reported that within an hour of leaving the clinic, AP ate an entire fried chicken sandwich at a fast food restaurant. Within a week, she had resumed her previous diet and she denied any difficulties swallowing or feeling as though food was "getting stuck." She regained all the weight she lost. In this case, performing VFSS prior to a clinical assessment would have exposed AP to unnecessary radiation and reinforced the idea that she was suffering from a serious illness. Acknowledging that her symptoms were real, giving her an explanation for those symptoms, and providing her with a safe environment and techniques to help her eat solid foods enabled her to overcome her fear of choking.

SUMMARY

Feeding problems in infants and young children are common. In otherwise healthy children who are developing and growing normally, feeding problems are usually not serious, are transient, and can be managed conservatively by reassuring the family, providing them with anticipatory guidance, and providing regular follow-up. A majority of more serious childhood feeding problems occur in children who have other medical, developmental, or behavioral problems. These more serious problems are best evaluated and treated by an interprofessional team who can identify and address issues in a child's medical and/or developmental history, problems with oral motor control and function, problems with swallowing, and behavioral and/or sensory issues that may interfere with normal feeding progression.

REFERENCES

1. Miller CK. Updates on pediatric feeding and swallowing problems. Curr Opin Otolaryngol Head Neck Surg 2009;17:194–9.
2. Phalen JA. Managing feeding problems and feeding disorders. Pediatr Rev 2013; 34:549–57.
3. Arts-Rodas D, Benoit D. Feeding problems in infancy and early childhood: identification and management. Paediatr Child Health 1998;3:21–7.
4. Ramasamy M, Perman JA. Pediatric feeding disorders. J Clin Gastroenterol 2000; 30:34–46.
5. Field D, Garland M, Williams K. Correlates of specific childhood feeding problems. J Paediatr Child Health 2003;39:299–304.
6. Rommel N, De Meyer AM, Feenstra L, et al. The complexity of feeding problems in 700 infants and young children presenting to a tertiary care institution. J Pediatr Gastroenterol Nutr 2003;37:75–84.
7. Kerzner B, Milano K, MacLean WC, et al. A practical approach to classifying and managing feeding difficulties. Pediatr 2015;135:344–53.
8. Rybak A. Organic and nonorganic feeding disorders. Ann Nutr Metab 2015; 66(Suppl 5):16–22.
9. Cano SC, Tiemeier H, Van Hoeken D, et al. Trajectories of picky eating during childhood: a general population study. Int J Eat Disord 2015;48:570–9.
10. Mathisen B, Worrall L, Masel J, et al. Feeding problems in in fants with gastro-oesophageal reflux disease: a controlled study. J Paediatr Child Health 1999; 35:163–9.
11. Nelson SP, Chen EH, Syniar GM, et al. One-year follow-up of symptoms of gastro-esophageal reflux during infancy. Pediatrics 1998;102:e67.
12. Dellert S, Hyams J, Tree W, et al. Feeding resistance and gastroesophageal reflux in infancy. J Pediatr Gastroenterol Nutr 1993;17:66–71.
13. Kerzner B. Clinical investigation of feeding difficulties in young children: a practical approach. Clin Pediatr 2009;48:960–5.
14. Chen IL, Gao WY, Johnson AP, et al. Proton pump inhibitor use in infants: FDA reviewer experience. J Pediatr Gastroenterol Nutr 2012;54:8–14.
15. Morris SE, Klein MD. Pre-feeding skills. 2nd edition. Tucson (AZ): Therapy Skill Builders; 2000.
16. Carruth BR, Ziegler PJ, Gordon A, et al. Developmental milestones and self-feeding behaviors in infants and toddlers. J Am Diet Assoc 2004; 104(1 Suppl 1):s51–6.
17. Beauchamp GK, Mennella J. Early flavor learning and its impact on later feeding behavior. J Pediatr Gastroenterol Nutr 2009;43:S25–30.
18. Beauchamp GK, Mennella J. Flavor perception in human infants: development and functional significance. Digestion 2011;83(Suppl 1):1–6.
19. Cooke LJ, Wardle J, Gibson EL, et al. Demographic, familial and trait predictors of fruit and vegetable consumption by preschool children. Public Health Nutr 2004;7:295–302.
20. Mennella J, Beauchamp GK. Developmental changes in the acceptance of protein hydrolysate formula. J Dev Behav Pediatr 1996;17:386–91.

21. Sellen DW. Evolution of infant and young child feeding: implications for contemporary public health. Annu Rev Nutr 2007;27:123–48.

22. AAP Section on Breastfeeding. Breastfeeding and the use of human milk. Pediatrics 2012;129(3):3827-e841.

23. American Academy of Family Physicians. Breastfeeding policy statement. 2007. Available at: www.aafp.org/online/en/home/policy/policies/b/breastfeedingpolicy.html. Accessed April 23, 2017.

24. Clayton HB, Li R, Perrine CG, et al. Prevalence and reasons for introducing infants early to solid foods: variation by milk feeding type. Pediatrics 2013;131: e1108–14.

25. Sellen DW. Comparison of infant feeding patterns reported for non-industrial populations with current recommendations. J Nutr 2001;131:2707–15.

26. Coulthard H, Harris G, Emmett P. Delayed introduction of lumpy foods to children during the complementary feeding period affects child's food acceptance and feeding at 7 years of age. Matern Child Nutr 2009;5:75–85.

27. Abrams EM, Greenhawt M, Fleischer DM, et al. Early solid food introduction: role in food allergy prevention and implications for breastfeeding. J Pediatr 2017;184: 13–8.

28. Carruth BR, Skinner JD. Feeding behaviors and other motor development in healthy children (2-24 months). J Am Coll Nutr 2002;21:88–96.

29. Gisel EG. Effect of food texture on the development of chewing of children between six months and two years of age. Dev Med Child Neurol 1991;33:69–79.

30. Wilson EM, Green JR, Weismer GA. A kinematic description of the temporal characteristics of jaw motion for early chewing: preliminary findings. J Speech Lang Hear Res 2012;55:626–38.

31. Logemann JA. Evaluation and treatment of swallowing disorders. 2nd edition. Austin (TX): Pro-Ed; 1998.

32. Reynolds J, Carroll S, Sturdivant C. Fiberoptic endoscopic evaluation of swallowing: a multidisciplinary alternative for assessment of infants with dysphagia in the neonatal intensive care unit. Adv Neonatal Care 2016;16:37–43.

33. Farneti D. Pooling score: and endoscopic model of evaluating severity of dysphagia. Acta Otorhinolaryngol Ital 2008;28:135–40.

34. Hiorns MP, Ryan MD. Current practice in paediatric videofluoroscopy. Pediatr Radiol 2006;36:911–9.

35. American Speech-Language-Hearing Association. Role of the speech-language pathologist in the performance and interpretation of endoscopic evaluation of swallowing: guidelines [Guidelines]. 2004. Available at: www.asha.org/policy. Accessed April 5, 2017.

36. Suterwala MS, Reynolds CS. Using fiberoptic endoscopic evaluation of swallowing to detect laryngeal penetration and aspiration in infants in the neonatal intensive care unit. J Perinatol 2017;37:404–8.

37. Weir KA, McMahan SM, Long G, et al. Radiation doses to children during modified barium swallow studies. Pediatr Radiol 2007;37:283–90.

38. Brenner D, Huda W. Effective dose: a useful concept in diagnostic radiology. Radiat Prot Dosimetry 2008;128:503–8.

39. American Speech-Language-Hearing Association (n. d). Pediatric Dysphagia. (Practice Portal). Available at: http://www.asha.org/Practice-Portal/Clinical-Topics/Pediatric-Dysphagia. Accessed April 24, 2017.

An Interprofessional Team Approach to the Differential Diagnosis of Children with Language Disorders

Xueman Lucy Liu, AuD/CCC-A/FAAA, MS/CCC-SLP[a],
Dawn M. Zahrt, PhD[b,c], Mark D. Simms, MD, MPH[b,c],*

KEYWORDS

- Interprofessional practice model • IPP model • Communication disorders
- Interdisciplinary diagnostic process

KEY POINTS

- Communication disorders may present with a wide range of symptoms and affect social, behavioral, emotional, and academic development.
- Speech and language difficulties may be isolated problems or a manifestation of a complex medical or psychological disorder.
- The interprofessional practice model provides a framework for professionals from multiple disciplines to work in a complementary manner to provide a comprehensive evaluation of children with communication disorders.

INTRODUCTION

The ability to understand and communicate with others is central to children's development. In the broadest sense, communication includes both verbal and nonverbal means. Delays or disruptions may have widespread consequences affecting academic, social, behavioral, and emotional function. Communication disorders in children may include isolated expressive language delay or errors of simple sound production (articulation), multiple sound production errors with some degree of motor planning deficits, or mixed expressive and receptive language delay with complex

Disclosure Statement: The authors have nothing to disclose.
[a] Bethel Hearing-Speaking Training Center, 7801 South Stemmons Freeway, Corinth, TX 76210, USA; [b] Section of Developmental Pediatrics, Department of Pediatrics, Medical College of Wisconsin, 8701 West Watertown Plank Road, Milwaukee, WI 53226, USA; [c] Child Development Center, Children's Hospital of Wisconsin, 13800 West North Avenue, Brookfield, WI 53005, USA
* Corresponding author.
E-mail address: msimms@mcw.edu

language processing difficulty. Physical anomalies, neurologic and genetic disorders, cognitive and intellectual disabilities, and emotional disturbances may contribute to communication disorders. In many instances, children who have difficulty understanding and using language at their age level may be misdiagnosed with intellectual impairment or with autism spectrum disorder (ASD). Making a differential diagnosis crosses many disciplines. Therefore, comprehensive evaluation may require an interprofessional approach and should include assessment of a child's speech and language abilities, physical and neurologic status, cognitive and emotional profile, and family history and social environment. This article describes the content and process of interprofessional assessment, and reviews the range of communication disorders commonly seen in children.

INTERPROFESSIONAL PRACTICE MODEL

Children with developmental disabilities often present with complex clinical problems. They frequently require the care of multiple medical subspecialists, psychologists, therapists, and educators to make accurate diagnoses and to provide appropriate and comprehensive services. For many patients and their families, obtaining and integrating the services needed is exhausting and confusing. Diagnostic confusion often arises when professionals from different disciplines approach the same problem with different conceptual frameworks and assumptions because each may use a variety of terms to describe the same phenomena. However, it has long been recognized that care is improved when professionals caring for a patient communicate and collaborate with each other.[1,2]

The interprofessional practice (IPP) model provides a framework for health care providers to work together to address the needs of patients and families.[3] The structure of these collaborations may vary depending on the particular setting and the nature and intensity of the patient's needs. An interprofessional team is composed of professionals with complementary skills who work together in a collaborative manner to provide comprehensive and coordinated care. For children with communication disorders, an interprofessional team should include, at a minimum, a speech-language pathologist, a pediatric psychologist, and a developmental pediatrician. If available and appropriate, other professionals may participate, including an audiologist, social worker, special education teacher, occupational therapist, physical therapist, and so forth (**Fig. 1**). Each member of the team brings a unique perspective and diagnostic framework and evaluates different aspects of the child's development. For young children, sequential evaluations on different days may ensure that the child is not fatigued; the order of the evaluations is not critical. Parents should participate in the evaluation process, and teachers and other caretakers should be asked to provide input and observations of the child in different settings. Although individual assessments are conducted independently, the team's members must meet to integrate the findings of each evaluation before meeting with the family. This is a shared decision-making process. Rather than simply listing individual findings, team members should integrate their findings and resolve any apparent discrepancies. Because all observations and findings represent a facet of the child's development and behavior, the final conclusions may reveal more than the results of any individual assessment.

GOALS OF AN INTERPROFESSIONAL EVALUATION

The first goal of an interprofessional team is to identify the child's profile of functional strengths and weaknesses. This profile provides critical information that may lead to

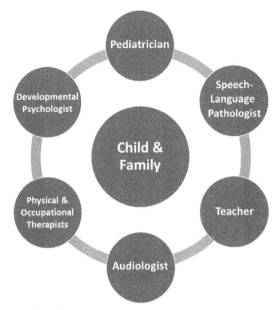

Fig. 1. The interprofessional team.

determining the child's principal and comorbid diagnoses. The ultimate goals of the evaluation are to help parents understand the nature of their child's difficulties, to recommend and prioritize strategies for guiding their child's development, to help parents and caregivers to understand the nature of their child's difficulties, and to help them to advocate appropriately for their child's needs.

SCOPE OF INDIVIDUAL DISCIPLINE ASSESSMENTS

The IPP model underscores the importance of evaluating a child's speech and language skills in the context of all factors that may affect a child's communication development (**Fig. 2**). Development of communication skills highly depends on the interaction of linguistic, cognitive, and physical abilities, and the language acquisition environment.

Speech and Language Evaluation

Communication encompasses all the ways in which words, sounds, signs, or behaviors to receive and express ideas, thoughts, and feelings are understood and used. An assessment begins at the broad level of verbal and nonverbal communication skills, addresses various facets of language development, and then evaluates speech sound production. Communication skills can be assessed even before children can utter words because infants communicate through eye gaze, gestures (pointing), facial expressions, joint attention, turn taking, laughter, and body movements. These paralinguistic communication skills are precursors of later oral language abilities and may foreshadow symptoms of significant developmental disorders.

Language
Language is a form of communication using conventional, agreed-upon symbols that include spoken or written words, or signs. The 2 components of language

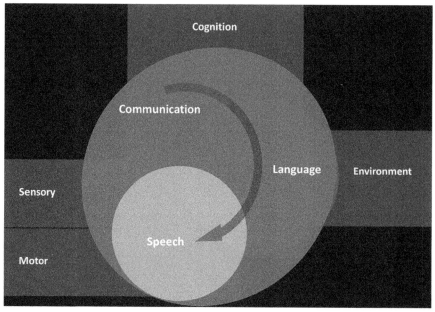

Fig. 2. Clinical framework for a comprehensive speech-language evaluation.

are receptive and expressive abilities. Language can be divided further into 5 domains[4]:

- Semantics refers to the meaning of words at all levels. For example, nouns, verbs, adjectives, adverbs, and prepositions are understood at the single word level. These same words may take on different meanings at the sentence or paragraph level.
- Syntax refers to the rules governing how words and phrases are arranged in the communication symbol system. Syntax skills emerge when children start to combine words.
- Morphology refers to how words and word stems are modified to indicate grammatical relationships. For example, plurals (book**s**), possessives (John**'s**), past tense (work**ed**), or adverbs (quick**ly**).
- Pragmatics refers to the ability to use verbal and nonverbal language appropriately to communicate effectively. These skills include initiating, joining, maintaining, and ending conversations; using appropriate words and expressions, forms of address; body posture, facial expressions, eye contact, and gestures; and understanding and using humor, sarcasm, metaphors, and so forth.
- Phonology refers to the rules of how sounds or minimal units of sign language are organized in the communication symbol system.

Formal evaluation with norm-referenced assessment tools can provide standard scores that compare a child's level of functioning with other children of the same age, and can also provide a profile of strengths and weaknesses in specific areas of communication.[5,6] **Box 1** lists commonly used tests of speech and language functioning suitable for preschool and school-age children (See Appendices 1 and 2 for test sources).

Box 1
Standardized speech and language assessment instruments

Parent report instruments

- Rossetti Infant-Toddler Language Scale
  - Age: birth to 3 years, 11 months

- Receptive-Expressive Emergent Language Test (REEL-3)
  - Age: birth to 3 years, 0 months

Expressive vocabulary tests

- Expressive Vocabulary Test (EVT-2)
  - Age: 2 years, 6 months to 90+ years

- Expressive One Word Picture Vocabulary Test (EOWPVT-4)
  - Age: 2 years, 0 months to 80+ years

- Structured Photographic Expressive Language Test (SPELT-P2)
  - Age: 3 years, 0 months to 5 years, 11 months

Receptive vocabulary tests

- Peabody Picture Vocabulary Test (PPVT-4)
  - Age: 2 years, 6 months to 90+ years

- Receptive One Word Picture Vocabulary Test (ROWPVT-4)
  - Age: 2 years, 0 months to 80+ years

Tests of language development

- Preschool Language Scale (PLS-5)
  - Age: birth to 7 years, 11 months

- Test of Early Language Development (TELD-3)
  - Age: 2 years, 0 months to 7 years, 11 months

- Clinical Evaluation of Language Fundamentals (CELF-P:2)
  - Age: 3 years, 0 months to 6 years, 11 months

- Test of Language Development (TOLD-4)
  - P-4 Age: 4 years, 0 months to 8 years, 11 months
  - I-4 Age: 8 years, 0 months to 17 years, 11 months

- Sequenced Inventory of Communication Development (SICD-R)
  - Age: 0 years, 4 months to 4 years, 0 months

- Test of Narrative Language (TNL-2)
  - Age: 5 years, 0 months to 15 years, 11 months

- Language Processing Test (LPT-3)
  - Age: 5 years, 0 months to 11 years, 11 months (exception: the Multiple Meanings subtests should not be administered to 5 years, 0 months–5 years, 11 months)

- Test of Auditory Comprehension of Language (TACL-4)
  - Age: 3 years, 0 months to 12 years, 11 months

- Comprehensive Assessment of Spoken Language (CASL-2)
  - Age: 3 years, 0 months to 21 years, 11 months

Tests of speech articulation and phonology

- Goldman Fristoe Test of Articulation (GFTA-2)
  - Age: 2 years, 0 months to 21 years, 11 months

- Clinical Assessment of Articulation and Phonology (CAAP-2)
  - Age: 2 years, 6 months to 11 years, 11 months

- Fisher-Logemann Test of Articulation Competence
  - Age: 3 years, 0 months to adult

- Photo Articulation Test (PAT-3)
  - Age: 3 years, 0 months to 8 years, 11 months

In addition to using norm-referenced standardized assessments, speech-language pathologists typically also collect and analyze language samples and conduct other forms of informal assessments when evaluating children's communication abilities. Observations during low-structure activities, such as free play, reveal important information regarding the length, complexity, coherence, and fluency of the child's expressive utterances in conversation and how the child responds to comments and directions. The child's pragmatic skills, such as eye contact and use of nonverbal forms of communication, can also easily be studied in naturalistic settings. These observations may demonstrate complete or partial lack of comprehension of what is spoken.

The profile of a child's speech and language abilities may suggest possible communication disorder diagnoses. For example, delay in both expressive and receptive language abilities when nonverbal cognitive abilities are normal is characteristic of specific language impairment (SLI). Children with SLI are at high-risk for persisting language and learning difficulties as they progress through their school years and into adulthood. Children whose expressive abilities are delayed but receptive language is at age level may have isolated expressive language disorder, which generally has a favorable prognosis for normal speech and language development, as well as learning. Alternatively, a severe speech disorder may impair a child's ability to talk with others despite age-appropriate understanding of language.[7]

Speech

Speech refers to the processes related to word sound production. Principal components of speech include articulation (accuracy and clarity of produced sounds), voice (quality, pitch, or loudness), and fluency (rate or rhythm).

Articulation refers to the physical (motoric) act of producing the correct sounds that make up words. Articulation errors may be described as substitutions (inserting a sound for another), omissions, additions, or distortions. Speech intelligibility in young children is often due to immaturity in sound production (pronunciation). There is a typical age-related sequence to children's ability to pronounce certain sounds. Phonology refers to how the individual sound patterns are organized to produce words so they are perceived as distinct. Children with phonological speech disorders seem to use atypical processes to simplify words, and there is a consistent pattern to their sound distortions. Childhood apraxia of speech is a more complex disorder in which there is inconsistent coordination of motor speech patterns. Speech disorders may be developmental (due to immaturity), the result of sensory deficits (hearing loss), oral structural abnormalities (cleft palate, enlarged tonsils and/or adenoids), neuromuscular weakness (cerebral palsy), or motor planning deficits.

Voice disorders may result from physical changes to the larynx due to edema (inflammation), nodules (from vocal misuse), or neurologic dysfunction (paralysis or spasm of the vocal folds).

Disfluency (breaks in the flow of speech) may be seen in otherwise typically developing children between age 2 and 5 years. This problem is thought to be related to the rapid development of language, particularly as children begin to use longer, more complex utterances. These disfluencies decrease as children develop greater proficiency in language. Stuttering is a neurodevelopmental speech disorder characterized by the repetition of sounds, syllables, or words, the prolongation of sounds, and/or speech that is stopped or blocked. It is estimated that 8% of children have a stuttering problem and most will recover without treatment. Recovery is less likely for children with a family history of stuttering, and in those who have been stuttering for more than a year. Persistent stuttering can have a significant impact on the person's ability to communicate and affect school, work, and social interactions. Cluttering refers to disfluency characterized by abnormally rapid and/or irregular speech. There may be accompanying language and phonological errors, as well as attention deficits. Cluttering may affect organization of thoughts, writing, and conversation.

Speech evaluation includes an examination of the oral mechanism to assess oropharyngeal structures (dental occlusion, tooth deviations, or integrity of the hard and soft palates) and muscle movement (speed, strength, range of movement, accuracy, coordination, and dissociation of lips, jaw, tongue, and velum). Speech sound evaluation includes a comprehensive error inventory, a pattern evaluation (both at the single word level and at the connected speech level), appraisal of stimulability (ability to correctly imitate speech sounds), and a speech perception assessment.

Feeding and swallowing
Children with neurodevelopmental delay or disorder often have feeding and swallowing difficulty. Evaluation involves direct observation of sucking, biting, chewing, and swallowing during feedings, and use of instrumentation, such as videofluoroscopy, to assess swallowing.[8-11]

Augmentative and alternative communication
Children with severe speech and language disorders may have very limited oral output and may benefit from augmentative and alternative communication (AAC) systems. This may take the form of a simple communication board with pictures, or an electronic device with functional, high-frequency words and phrases that can be spoken electronically. The choice of ACC system is based on the child's physical, communicative, linguistic, and intellectual capabilities, and by the child's environment and typical communicative situations and partners.

Psychological Evaluation

Psychological evaluations of children with communication disorders encompass multiple areas of function that affect, and are affected by, language, including intellectual ability; emotional, social, and behavioral development; and academic functioning.

Intellectual ability
Intellectual ability plays a large role in language development and delay in communication skills is among first signs of intellectual disability (ID) in young children. Of children who fail a screen for language development, approximately one-third have generalized (verbal and nonverbal) cognitive delay.[12] In contrast, children with SLI have age-appropriate nonverbal cognitive abilities. A comprehensive psychological evaluation is needed to distinguish between ID and SLI. Additionally, the prognosis for children with all types of communication delays correlates highly with cognitive ability. More specifically, those with strong nonverbal cognitive abilities are generally better able to compensate for communication difficulties. Thus, assessing the intellectual ability of children with communication delays is important for both differential diagnosis and prognosis.

It is often not appreciated that many standardized cognitive assessment instruments rely heavily on a child's language skills because they are administered using verbal directives and require verbal responses from the child. Even tasks that do not require a verbal response from the child, and are therefore often considered to reflect nonverbal abilities, are frequently administered verbally and require receptive language skills. As a result, these test instruments may provide inaccurate assessments and can result in a misdiagnosis in a child with language impairment.

Several valid nonverbal test measures are available to evaluate children with communication disorders (**Table 1**). The items are administered with nonverbal directives (eg, gestures, demonstration) and the child responds nonverbally. It should be noted, however, that these measures depend on the child's cooperation and fine motor skills.

A diagnosis of a language disorder may still be appropriate in children with generalized cognitive delays if a significant discrepancy exists between verbal and nonverbal abilities.

Importance of behavioral observations and informal assessment

Administering a standardized test measure to assess intellectual ability is an important part of diagnostic evaluation of children with communication challenges. Results from this testing can aid in differential diagnosis and assist in identifying the child's strengths and weaknesses. However, a test score should never be interpreted in isolation. Rather, it is essential that such scores be considered in combination with other observations made during the evaluation. Key factors or behaviors to watch for during administration of testing include cooperation, participation, effort, attention, and activity level. It is also important to observe the child's reactions to being challenged and having to follow adult-directed activities. Whether or not test scores should be considered a reasonable estimate of a child's ability and functioning depends on these observations.

In a broader sense, observing a child's interactions with their parents during an evaluation can also add to the assessment process, as can taking note of the child's interactions with the psychologist. Specific questions to consider when observing the child's interactions include

- Does the child bring toys to show the adults in the room?
- Does the child look to see if the adults in the room are watching their test performance?
- How does the child react when praised?
- Can the child be easily engaged in play?
- How does the child react if language demands are removed from play situations?

Table 1
Nonverbal cognitive assessment instruments

Instrument	Age Range	Administration Directions
Merrill-Palmer-Revised: Scales of Development	1 mo–6 y, 5 mo	Predominantly nonverbal with verbal directives for some items
Central Institute for the Deaf Preschool Performance Scale	2 y–5 y, 5 mo	Nonverbal, with optional verbal cues
Leiter International Performance Scale, 3rd edition	3–75+ y	Nonverbal
Primary Test of Nonverbal Intelligence	3 y–9 y, 11 mo	Minimal verbal directives
Universal Nonverbal Intelligence Test, 2nd edition	5 y–21 y, 11 mo	Nonverbal
Comprehensive Test of Nonverbal Intelligence, 2nd edition	6 y–89 y, 11 mo	Nonverbal, with optional verbal directives
Test of Nonverbal Intelligence, 4th edition	6 y–89 y, 11 mo	Nonverbal, with optional verbal directives

Additionally, it is valuable to observe the children's play in terms of what types of toys they seek out on their own and how they play with them. Questions to ask when observing the child during play include

- Does the child play in an organized fashion?
- Does the child play with the toys in an appropriate manner?
- Does the child show evidence of make-believe and pretend play?
- Does the child sustain attention with a toy for a period of time or switch frequently between toys?

It is also beneficial to observe whether the child plays independently and/or whether she or he tries to engage the adults in their play. Children's emotional reactions during their evaluations are also important to take note of, particularly in terms of transition between activities, and their reactions when denied their way or when something does not go according to their wishes. All of these observations can aid in differential diagnosis as it pertains to the children's social, emotional, and behavioral functioning. For instance, a child who sustains attention well during nonverbal testing and play is unlikely to have a primary attention deficit.

Emotional, social, and behavioral development

Inability to communicate effectively usually has a profound influence on children's emotional, social, and behavioral development.[13] Surveys of children with language impairment have repeatedly noted a high rate of associated emotional and behavioral disorders.[14,15] Among children seen in mental health clinics for emotional and behavioral concerns, approximately half also have significant, and often previously unrecognized, language impairments.[16] In turn, children with behavioral and social-emotional disorders may have difficulty communicating with others despite typical development of basic language abilities.

Anxiety disorder and selective mutism

Anxiety disorders are very common in children and adolescents.[17] Symptoms include difficulty with emotional regulation, irritability, behavioral inhibition, social avoidance, and poor ability to adapt to change. Children overwhelmed with anxiety may experience difficulty communicating effectively. Selective mutism is a relatively uncommon form of social anxiety in which an individual fails to speak in certain situations even though they can speak without issue in other situations, typically at home and with parents and close family members.[18] Children with selective mutism are often reported to have normal language abilities. The situational nature of the communication difficulty seen in anxiety disorder distinguishes it from a global communication disorder.

Autism spectrum disorder

Communication skills are essential to building social relationships. Deficits in social communication ability are a core feature of ASD. In contrast to other developmental disorders in which communication difficulty is found, individuals with ASD display little interest in interacting with others (ie, they lack a social drive); have difficulty interpreting the intentions and meanings of other people's behaviors (ie, they lack theory of mind); and demonstrate restricted, repetitive patterns of behavior, interests, or activities (RRBIs). In contrast, children who have a communication disorder but not a diagnosis of ASD exhibit a strong desire to socialize even though their communication skills are poor and they use nonverbal means of communication to compensate for verbal communication limitations. These children also lack RRBIs.[19]

Academic functioning

Children with communication disorders are at an increased risk for learning-related difficulties. In particular, language impairment during preschool years is highly associated with reading and writing difficulties during the school years. This, in turn, may lead to overall academic difficulties.

Medical Evaluation

The physician's role in the interprofessional evaluation process is to identify physical, neurologic, genetic, environmental, and/or chronic health factors that may affect a child's communication difficulties. Comprehensive medical history should include prenatal and birth events, developmental milestones, prior medical history, current health status, and family history. Physical examination should focus on relevant risk factors and medically diagnosable conditions. Any disorder affecting a child's development can affect speech and language development. Although not exhaustive, **Box 2** highlights some significant medical considerations.

Health history

Prenatal history may reveal medical complications or other factors that place the child at risk for a communication disorder. For example, polyhydramnios (excessive amniotic fluid) may be the result of a structural or neurologic disorder that impairs the oral-motor function of a fetus. Prematurely born infants may experience neurodevelopmental delays even if they did not encounter any significant medical complications in the perinatal period.[20] Term infants with symptoms of neonatal encephalopathy, seizures, or intrauterine growth restriction (birth weight less than the tenth percentile for gestational age) are at increased risk of neurodevelopmental disabilities that include speech and language disorders.[21] In the postpartum period, prolonged feeding difficulties may be associated with oral-motor coordination problems that may affect speech in the future. Chronic illness of any type, particularly if it results in repeated hospitalization or poor physical growth, may affect language development. Recurrent seizures are often associated with developmental and communication disorders. Sequelae of severe traumatic brain injury may include speech, language, and swallowing problems.[22] Of note, recurrent ear infections are not strongly associated with subsequent delays in language development.[23,24]

Careful review of family history for individuals who were late talkers or had reading or learning disorders is very important because disorders of speech and language often have a strong genetic component.[25] Delay in achieving early developmental milestones, particularly early social, gestural, or linguistic skills, may be the first signs of a communication disorder.

At any age, a clear history of developmental regression should raise concern and prompt further investigation of possible autism, metabolic storage disorders (mucopolysaccharidosis, Batten disease), Rett syndrome, or epilepsy syndromes.

Physical examination

Physical examination may reveal signs of dysmorphic features suggestive of craniofacial disorder, congenital malformation, or genetic syndrome associated with developmental delay.

Craniofacial disorders are structural anomalies of the face, ears, and neck that are usually obvious at the time of birth. Cleft palate may be either an isolated finding or associated with a recognizable syndrome. Bifid uvula, caused by a submucous cleft palate, is often missed during postpartum and well-baby examinations if there are no other symptoms (feeding or nasal regurgitation)[26–28] and may result in impaired speech development. Pierre-Robin deformation sequence (mandibular anomaly with

Box 2
Medical correlates with communication disorders

Prenatal factors

- Intrauterine growth restriction
- Decreased fetal movement pattern
- Polyhydramnios
- Exposure to drugs, toxins, infections, and so forth

Perinatal factors

- Prematurity with or without obvious central nervous system (CNS) complications
  - Intraventricular hemorrhage
  - Bronchopulmonary dysplasia
- Term with neonatal encephalopathy, CNS complications
- Early or persistent oral-motor feeding difficulty

Postnatal factors

- Poor physical growth (failure to thrive)
- Traumatic brain injury
- Hearing deficit

Causes of developmental regression

- Autism
- Rett syndrome
- Epilepsy (Landau-Kleffner syndrome)
- Metabolic storage disease (eg, mucopolysaccharidosis)

Craniofacial anomalies

- Pierre Robin deformation
- Syndromes associated with cleft palate: Stickler syndrome, velocardiofacial syndrome, Treacher Collins syndrome
- Microcephaly
- Macrocephaly

Genetic syndromes

- Fragile X syndrome, Williams syndrome, Down syndrome

Neurologic disorders

- Congenital anomalies of brain
- Hypertonia or cerebral palsy
- Hypotonia, congenital myopathy, Prader-Willi (15q11–13) syndrome, Williams (7q11.23) syndrome, Phelan-McDermid (22q13) syndrome, or Down (trisomy 21) syndrome
- Metabolic disorders
  - Cerebral creatine deficiency syndromes
    - Guanidinoacetate n-methyl transferase deficiency (GAMT)
    - Arginine: glycine amidinotransferase deficiency (AGAT)
    - Cerebral creatine transporter deficiency (SLC6A8)
  - Lysosomal storage diseases
    - Mucopolysaccharidoses
    - Tay-Sachs disease
    - Neuronal ceroid lipofuscinosis (Batten disease)
    - Niemann-Pick disease
    - Metachromatic leukodystrophy
    - Niemann-Pick disease
    - Stroke or traumatic brain injury

micrognathia, large tongue, and a U-shaped cleft palate) is often associated with a multisystem genetic syndrome.[29]

Abnormalities of physical growth may reflect an underlying disease process that can affect development. Poor growth (failure-to-thrive) may be caused by genetic disorders (Prader-Willi syndrome), chronic illness, environmental understimulation or neglect, and physical abuse. Microcephaly (head circumference <2 standard deviations for age) can result from any factor that interferes with brain growth and is associated with cerebral malformations, brain injuries from intrauterine infection, hypoxic-ischemic encephalopathy, intraventricular or intracerebral bleeding, subdural hematoma, stroke, genetic, or metabolic disorders.[30,31] Macrocephaly (head circumference >2 standard deviations for age) may be a benign familial trait, or result from autism, hydrocephalus, cerebral overgrowth (Soto syndrome, Weaver syndrome, or Beckwith-Wiedemann syndrome), metabolic disorders (creatine deficiency syndromes or lysosomal storage diseases), or bone dysplasia (achondroplasia).[32]

Neurologic examination

Neurologic examination may reveal abnormalities of muscle tone and or strength. Hypertonia (high resting muscle tone) is typical of injury to the motor cortex of the brain (cerebral palsy), and may result in problems with feeding and swallowing (dysphagia) and speech articulation (dysarthria). Hypotonia (low resting muscle tone) is common in children with global developmental delay, congenital myopathy, and in certain genetic disorders. Mild benign congenital hypotonia is also frequently noted in children with SLI.[33]

Inborn errors of metabolism are relatively rare but may be associated with global developmental delay, epilepsy, or regression in development. Although very rare, speech delay is among prominent symptoms in cerebral creatine deficiency, and treatment may result in improvement of clinical symptoms.[34,35]

Epilepsy is often associated with cognitive impairment and language disorder.[36,37] The most common form of childhood epilepsy, so-called benign rolandic epilepsy, is associated with expressive and receptive language difficulty, phonological processing weakness, and reading difficulty.[38] Landau-Kleffner syndrome (acquired epileptic aphasia) begins between ages 3 and 7 years and presents as a sudden or gradual loss of language abilities.[39]

Medical diagnostic testing

Unless there is a suggestion of a specific underlying cause (eg, abnormal physical or neurologic examination, ID, autism, regression in development, or seizure disorder), medical diagnostic tests are not usually indicated in children with delayed speech or language development.

Despite strong evidence that language disorders have a genetic basis, no specific chromosomal anomalies have been identified to assist with or to confirm the diagnosis. Several studies have noted an increased rate of structural brain abnormalities in MRIs of normally intelligent children with isolated language impairment. However, findings were inconsistent, did not correlate with severity, and did not help with treatment or prognosis.[40,41] Similarly, electroencephalography (EEG) studies are abnormal in about one-third of patients with SLI without clinical seizures, but there is no correlation between the severity of the language deficit and the extent of EEG abnormalities, and no evidence that treating these EEG findings with medication improves the language development.[42]

INTERPROFESSIONAL DIAGNOSTIC PROCESS

Visits for evaluations should be scheduled to accommodate the needs of the child and family. To avoid fatigue, assessments should be limited to 1 per day. However, this can be modified if parental work schedules or travel distance present a burden for the family.

Once the evaluations have been completed, clinicians should confer to resolve any discrepant findings before meeting with the parents to discuss their diagnoses. Diagnostic considerations should be discussed in light of the child's and the family's presenting complaints and developmental history. It is important to recognize that developmental diagnoses may be functional and/or etiologic. At a minimum, the team should be able to arrive at descriptive diagnoses based on the child's clinical characteristics and profile of developmental strengths and weaknesses. Functional diagnoses are defined by their specific clinical characteristics (eg, cognitive impairment, language impairment, ASD, anxiety disorder, or attention deficit-hyperactivity disorder [ADHD]). A mismatch between children's abilities and what they are expected to do or learn may result in behavioral or emotional reactions that complicate the clinical picture. In most cases, an accurate descriptive diagnosis leads to effective strategies to improve functional use of language, and may suggest possible psychological or medical treatments for associated symptoms (ADHD, anxiety, or depression). Etiologic diagnoses address the underlying causes of the problems (eg, a specific genetic abnormality or brain malformation or injury) and may or may not have a direct impact on treatment strategies. In some very rare cases, medical therapies may improve communication abilities. However, even if a condition cannot be cured, an established etiologic diagnosis can provide useful information regarding prognosis and risk of recurrence.

Assessment of preschool age children may be particularly challenging due to behaviors that interfere with the evaluation itself. As a result, it may be difficult to arrive at firm conclusions regarding specific diagnoses in this age range. For example, a child may react differently on different days and in response to different challenges, settings, and individuals. Through a group process of synthesizing individual data, an interdisciplinary team may arrive at a diagnosis that transcends each individual discipline's findings. It is also acceptable to conclude that certain aspects of the child's development may remain unexplained despite the team's best efforts. Thus, diagnostic conclusions and treatment recommendations should be based on a combination of parental history and clinical observations that are tempered by the results of structured evaluations.

Parent Counseling

The final, and most important, step in the IPP model takes place when the team meets with the parents to review their findings and to offer recommendations for continued care. It is the authors' practice to allow approximately 1 hour for these visits, and to encourage parents to invite any other individuals they wish to join them at this meeting (eg, grandparents, teachers, or therapists), The goal is to avoid technical jargon and to present the findings in lay terms. It is particularly important to explain how the team members have used their findings to arrive at their diagnoses and recommendations. It is also important to share with parents those aspects of the child's problems that were not fully explained during the evaluation process. Typically, if parents have been given the opportunity to participate in the evaluation process, most of the parent counseling meeting will focus on choosing the next steps for treatments and monitoring.

CHALLENGES OF THE INTERPROFESSIONAL PROCESS

Professionals are typically educated in the theoretic frameworks, scientific bases, terminology, and practices of their specific discipline. Training experiences may not

---

Box 3
Barriers to effective interprofessional practice

- Insufficient time allotted for face-to-face team meetings and for all members to meet with the family
- Lack of clearly defined roles and responsibilities for each team member in the interdisciplinary evaluation process
- Failure to develop common language and shared conceptual frameworks to explain developmental processes and disorders
- Frequent rotation of members on and off a given team may delay the achievement of this goal.

---

include practicing in an interprofessional setting, and professionals may not feel comfortable collaborating with other disciplines regarding diagnoses or treatment recommendations. Team members in an interprofessional setting need to be flexible and learn to appreciate diverse ways of understanding the same problem, to value others' perspectives, and to develop a common language so that parents and caretakers receive a coherent explanation for their child's problems and the basis for the team's treatment recommendations.[43] This process takes time and experience working together. It is facilitated by a strong leader who ensures and values equal participation of all team members. Over time, interprofessional teams become more effective as members learn from each other and develop common approaches to working in a collaborative manner with families.

The IPP model also requires organizational and financial support for time that may not be reimbursable under typical fee-for-service programs. For example, team meetings in which members meet face-to-face to review and integrate their findings is currently not a billable service.[44] Additional factors that may detract from effective team functioning are noted in **Box 3**.

SUMMARY

A coordinated interprofessional team evaluation is generally more efficient than the more typical series of individual subspecialty evaluations because this allows team members to share common background information and focus on their individual areas of expertise. The clinical picture that emerges from this process often extends beyond the scope of any single professional discipline. Parents who receive coherent explanations and recommendations are better able to prioritize their treatment options. They feel more confident in their decisions and are better advocates for their children. For professionals, the benefits of working in an interprofessional setting include expanding their knowledge and learning from colleagues.

REFERENCES

1. Parrish RA, Oppenheimer S. The interdisciplinary team approach. In: Wolraich ML, Drotar DD, Dworkin PH, et al, editors. Developmental-behavioral pediatrics: evidence and practice. 1st edition. Philadelphia: Mosby Elsevier; 2008. p. 203–14.
2. Institute of Medicine Committee on Quality of Health Care in America. Crossing the quality chasm: a new health system for the 21st century. Washington, DC: National Academy Press; 2001.

3. Patel DR, Pratt HD, Patel ND. Team processes and team care for children with developmental disabilities. Pediatr Clin North America 2008;55:1375–90.
4. Gleason JB. The development of language. 6th edition. Boston: Pearson Education, Inc; 2005.
5. McCauley RJ, Swisher L. Psychometric review of language and articulation tests for preschool children. J Speech Hear Dis 1984;49:34–42.
6. Plante E, Vance R. Selection of preschool language tests: a data-based approach. Lang Speech Hear Serv Sch 1994;25:15–24.
7. Simms M. Language disorders in children: classification and clinical syndromes. Pediatr Clin N Am 2007;54:437–67.
8. American Speech-Language-Hearing Association. Position statement and guidelines for instrumental diagnostic procedures for swallowing. Am J Speech Lang Path 1992;34(Suppl 7):25–33.
9. Logemann JA. Evaluation and treatment of swallowing disorders. Austin: Pro-Ed; 1998.
10. Arvedson JC, Lefton-Grief MA. Pediatric videofluoroscopic swallow studies: a professional manual with caregiver guidelines. San Antonio: Communication Skill Builders, Psychological Corp; 1998.
11. American Speech-Language-Hearing Association. Roles of speech-language pathologists in swallowing and feeding disorders: technical report. https://doi.org/10.1044/policy.TR2001-00150.
12. Stevenson J, Richman N. The prevalence of language delay in population of three-year-old children and its association of general retardation. Dev Med Child Neuro 1976;18:431–41.
13. Im-Bolter N, Cohen NJ. Language impairment and psychiatric comorbidities. Pediatr Clin N Am 2007;54:525–42.
14. Cantwell DP, Baker L. Psychiatric and developmental disorders in children with communication disorders. Washington, DC: American Psychiatric Press; 1991.
15. Beitchman JH, Hood J, Rochon J, et al. Empirical classification of speech/language impairment in children: II. Behavioral characteristics. J Am Acad Child Adolesc Psychiatry 1989;28:118–23.
16. Cohen NJ, Davine M, Horodeszky N, et al. Unsuspected language impairment in psychiatrically disturbed children: prevalence and language and behavioral characteristics. J Am Acad Child Adolesc Psychiatry 1993;32:595–603.
17. Beesdo K, Knappe S, Pine DS. Anxiety and anxiety disorders in children and adolescents: developmental issues and implications for DSM-V. Pediatr Clin N Am 2009;32:483–524.
18. Viana AG, Beidel DC, Rabian B. Selective mutism: a review and integration of the last 15 years. Clin Psychol Rev 2009;29:57–67.
19. Simms M. When autistic behavior suggests a disease other than classic autism. Pediatr Clin N Am 2017;64:127–38.
20. Aram D, Hack M, Hawkins S, et al. Very low birthweight children and speech and language development. J Speech Hear Res 1991;34:1169–79.
21. Geva R, Eshel R, Leitner Y, et al. Neuropsychological outcome of children with intrauterine growth restriction: a 9-year prospective study. Pediatrics 2006;118:91–100.
22. Ylvisaker M. Communication outcome following traumatic brain injury. Semin Speech Lang 1992;13:239–50.
23. Roberts JE, Rosenfeld RM, Zeisel SA. Otitis media and speech and language: a meta-analysis of prospective studies. Pediatrics 2004;113:e238–48.

24. Paradise JL, Dollaghan CA, Campbell TF, et al. Language, speech sound production, and cognition in three-year-old children in relation to otitis media in their first three years of life. Pediatrics 2000;105:1119–30.
25. Hayiou-Thomas ME. Genetic and environmental influences on early speech, language and literacy development. J Commun Disord 2008;41:397–408.
26. Oji T, Sakamoto Y, Ogata H, et al. A 25-year review of cases with submucous cleft palate. Int J Pediatr Otorhinolaryngol 2013;77:1183–5.
27. Reiter R, Brosch S, Wefel H, et al. The submucous cleft palate: diagnosis and therapy. Int J Pediatr Otorhinolaryngol 2011;75:85–8.
28. ten Dam E, van der Heiden P, Korsten-Meijer AG, et al. Age of diagnosis and evaluation of consequence of submucous cleft palate. Int J Pediatr Otorhinolaryngol 2013;77:1019–24.
29. Shprintzen RJ. Pierre Robin, micrognathia, and airway obstruction: the dependency of treatment on accurate diagnosis. Int Anesthesiology Clin 1988;26: 64–71.
30. Aggarwal A, Mittal H, Patil R, et al. Clinical profile of children with developmental delay and microcephaly. J Neurosci Rural Pract 2013;4:288–91.
31. Ashwal S, Michelson D, Plawner L, et al. Practice parameter: evaluation of the child with microcephaly (an evidence-based review): report of the quality standards subcommittee of the American Academy of Neurology and the Practice Committee of the Child Neurology Society. Neurology 2009;73:887–97.
32. Williams CA, Dagli A, Battaglia A. Genetic disorders associated with macrocephaly. Am J Med Genet A 2008;146A:2023–37.
33. Powell RP, Bishop DV. Clumsiness and perceptual problems in children with specific language impairment. Dev Med Child Neuro 1992;34:755–65.
34. Stockler-Ipsiroglu S, van Karnebeek CD. Cerebral creatine deficiencies: a group of treatable intellectual developmental disorders. Semin Neurol 2014;34:350–6.
35. Iqbal F. Human guanidinoacetate n-methyl transferase (GAMT) deficiency: a treatable inborn error of metabolism. Pak J Pharm Sci 2015;28:2207–11.
36. Selassie GR, Viggedal G, Olsson I, et al. Speech, language, and cognition in preschool children with epilepsy. Dev Med Child Neuro 2008;50:432–8.
37. Parkinson GM. High incidence of language disorder in children with focal epilepsies. Dev Med Child Neuro 2002;44:533–7.
38. Smith AB, Bajomo O, Pal DK. A meta-analysis of literacy and language in children with rolandic epilepsy. Dev Med Child Neuro 2015;57:1019–26.
39. Stefanatos G. Changing perspectives on Landau-Kleffner syndrome. Clin Neuropsychol 2011;25:963–88.
40. Trauner D, Wulfeck B, Tallal P, et al. Neurological and MRI profiles of children with developmental language impairment. Dev Med Child Neuro 2000;42:470–5.
41. Webster RI, Erdos C, Evans K, et al. Neurological and magnetic resonance imaging findings in children with developmental language impairment. J Child Neuro 2008;23:870–7.
42. Venkateswaran S, Shevell M. The case against routine electroencephalography in specific language impairment. Pediatrics 2008;122:e911–6.
43. Pearson PH. The interdisciplinary team process, or the professionals' tower of babel. Developmental Med Child Neurol 1983;25:390–5.
44. Virani T. Interprofessional collaborative teams. 2012; Canadian Health Services Research Foundation. Available at: http://www.cfhi-fcass.ca/sf-docs/default-source/commissioned-research-reports/Virani-Interprofessional-EN.pdf?sfvrsn=0. Accessed May 18, 2017.

APPENDIX 1: PSYCHOLOGICAL TEST SOURCES (ASSESSMENT INSTRUMENTS)

Merrill-Palmer-Revised Scales of Development (M-P-R)
- Roid G, Sampers J. Merrill-Palmer-revised scales of development. Wood Dale, IL: C H Stoelting Co; 2004.

Central Institute for the Deaf Preschool Performance Scale (CID-PPS)
- Geers A, Lane H. Central Institute for the Deaf preschool performance scale. Chicago: C H Stoelting Co; 1984.

Leiter international performance scale (Leiter 3)
- Roid GH, Miller LJ. Leiter international performance scale. 3rd edition. Wood Dale, IL: C H Stoelting Co; 2013.

Primary test of nonverbal intelligence (PTONI)
- Ehrler D, McGhee R. Primary test of nonverbal intelligence. Austin, TX: Pro-Ed; 2008.

Universal Nonverbal Intelligence Test (UNIT-2)
- Bracken BA, McCallum RS. Universal nonverbal intelligence test. 2nd edition. Austin, TX: Pro-Ed; 2016.

Comprehensive Test of Nonverbal Intelligence (CTONI-2)
- Hammill DD, Pearson NA, Wiederholt JL. Comprehensive test of nonverbal intelligence. 2nd edition. Austin, TX: Pro-Ed; 2009.

Test of nonverbal intelligence (TONI-4)
- Brown L, Sherbenou RJ, Johnsen SK. Test of nonverbal intelligence. 4th edition. Austin, TX: Pro-Ed; 2010.

APPENDIX 2: LANGUAGE TEST SOURCE (ASSESSMENT INSTRUMENTS)

Rossetti infant-toddler language scale
- Rossetti L. The Rossetti infant-toddler language scale. East Moline, IL: LinguiSystems; 2006.

Receptive-expressive emergent language test (REEL-3)
- Bzoch KR, League R, Brown V. Receptive-expressive emergent language test. 3rd edition. Austin, TX: Pro-Ed; 2003.

Expressive vocabulary test (EVT-2)
- Williams KT. Expressive vocabulary test. 2nd edition. Minneapolis, MN: Pearson; 2007.

Structured Photographic Expressive language test -Preschool 2 (SPELT-P-2)
- Dawson JI, Stout C, Eyer J, et al. Structured photographic expressive language test. 2nd edition. DeKalb, IL: Janelle Publications; 2005.

Peabody picture vocabulary test (PPVT-4)
- Dunn LM, Dunn DM. Peabody picture vocabulary test. 4th edition. Bloomington, MN: Pearson; 2007.

Receptive one word picture vocabulary test (ROWPVT-4)
- Brownell R. Receptive one-word picture vocabulary test. 4th edition. Novato, CA: Academic Therapy Publications; 2011.

Preschool language scale (PLS-5)
- Zimmerman IL, Steiner VG. Pond RE. Preschool language scales. 5th edition. Bloomington, MN: Pearson; 2011.

Test of early language development (TELD-3)
- Hresko W, Reid D, Hammill D. Test of early language development. 3rd edition. Austin, TX: Pro-Ed; 1999.

Clinical evaluation of language fundamentals-preschool 2 (CELF-P-2)
- Wiig EH, Secord WA, Semel E. Clinical evaluation of language fundamentals preschool. 2nd edition. San Antonio, TX: Harcourt Assessment, Inc; 2004.

Test of language development, primary (TOLD-P-4)
- Newcomer PL, Hammill DD. Test of language development, primary. 4th edition. Austin, TX: Pro-Ed; 2008.

Sequenced inventory of communication development, revised (SICD-R)
- Hedrick DL, Prather EM, Tobin AR. Sequenced inventory of communication development, revised. Seattle, WA: University of Washington Press; 1984.

Test of narrative language (TNL-2)
- Gillam RB, Pearson NA. Test of narrative language Austin, TX: Pro-Ed; 2017.

Language processing test (LPT-3)
- Richard G, Hanner M. Language processing test. East Moline, IL: LinguiSystems; 2005.

Test of auditory comprehension of language (TACL-4)
- Carrow-Woolfolk E. Test of auditory comprehension of language. Austin, TX: Pro-Ed; 2014.

Comprehensive assessment of spoken language (CASL-2)
- Carrow-Woolfolk E. Comprehensive assessment of spoken language. 2nd edition. Torrance, CA: Western Psychological Services; 2016.

Goldman-Fristoe test of articulation (GFTA-3)
- Goldman R, Fristoe M. Goldman-Fristoe test of articulation. 3rd edition. Bloomington, MN: Pearson; 2015.

Clinical assessment of articulation and phonology (CAAP-2)
- Secord W, Donohue JS. Clinical assessment of articulation and phonology. 2nd edition. Greenville, SC: Super Duper Publications; 2014.

Fisher-Logemann test of articulation competence
- Fisher H, Logemann J. Fisher-Logemann test of articulation competence. Boston: Houghton Mifflin; 1971.

Photo articulation test (PAT-3)
- Lippke BA, Dickey SE, Selmar JW, et al. Photo articulation test. Austin, TX: Pro-Ed; 1997.

Open Up and Let Us In

An Interprofessional Approach to Oral Health

Mona M. Sedrak, PhD, PA[a],*, Laura M. Doss, DDS[b,1]

KEYWORDS

• Oral health • Interprofessional • Primary care • Dental caries

KEY POINTS

• Dental caries is the single most common chronic disease of childhood in the United States.
• Health care providers who care for children must embrace a shared responsibility for children's oral health and work interprofessionally to overcome the separation between dentistry and medicine.
• Access to dental care is one of the barriers to improved oral health for children.
• Primary care providers who care for children already have an established role in prevention and early identification of health problems; thus they are ideal front-line providers who can detect oral health discrepancies and begin the process of care and prevention.

INTRODUCTION

Dental caries is the single most common chronic disease of childhood in the United States. Approximately 1 in 5 (20%) children, 5 to 11 years of age, and 1 in 7 (13%) adolescents, 12 to 19 years of age, have at least one untreated decayed tooth.[1,2] Children from low socioeconomic families and African American decent are at increased risk for experiencing dental decay. In 2009 to 2010, 1 in 4 children aged 3 to 5 years living in poverty experienced untreated caries, 2.5 times that of other children.[1,2]

Untreated dental conditions contribute to poor overall health, dysfunctional speech production, and poor nutrition.[3–6] Children experiencing early childhood caries (ECC) may experience pain with eating, and thus, they are often underweight.[7] Nutritional deficiencies during childhood can negatively impact cognitive development.[8] Children with poor oral and overall health are 2.3 times more likely to demonstrate poor school

Disclosure Statement: The authors have nothing to disclose.
[a] Seton Hall University, School of Health and Medical Sciences, 400 South Orange Avenue, South Orange, NJ, 07079 USA; [b] Elizabeth Mueller and Associates, The Pediatric Dental Center, 6396 Thornberry Ct, Mason, OH 45040, USA
[1] Present address: 8318 Turtlecreek Lane, Montgomery, OH 45242.
* Corresponding author. 167 Forest Lake Drive N, Andover, NJ 07821.
E-mail address: Mona.Sedrak@Shu.Edu

Pediatr Clin N Am 65 (2018) 91–103
https://doi.org/10.1016/j.pcl.2017.08.023
0031-3955/18/© 2017 Elsevier Inc. All rights reserved.
pediatric.theclinics.com

performance.[9] Up to 52 million school hours are lost annually as a result of dental problems.[5] Self-image, self-esteem, and self-confidence can also be deeply affected by poor oral hygiene and can affect the developing psyche of children, with life-long consequences in social, educational, and occupational environments.[10,11]

Despite improvements over the past 2 decades in US children's oral health, the silent epidemic of untreated oral diseases continues.[12,13] Although Medicaid provides dental services, only 33% to 57% of eligible children receive preventive or restorative dental services.[14–16] Rather than using the preventative dental coverage that Medicaid provides, emergency departments are being used to address dental pain and infections. Increasing visits to the Emergency Department is in part due to a shortage of dentists who accept Medicaid and treat children.[14–16] Pediatricians, nurse practitioners, physician assistants, speech-language pathologists, and other health professionals who care for children must embrace a shared responsibility for children's oral health, and work interprofessionally to overcome the separation between dentistry and medicine.

EARLY CHILDHOOD CARIES

Dental caries is a nonclassic infectious disease that results from a complex interaction between oral flora and dietary carbohydrates on the tooth surface. The development of caries is a process that starts with a carious lesion appearing as an opaque white spot on enamel (**Fig. 1**). The white spot lesion occurs as a result of increased bacterial load and frequency of carbohydrate consumption. Progressive demineralization of a white spot lesion results in a cavitation of the enamel, with eventual loss of supported tooth structure, resulting in a dental cavity (**Fig. 2**).

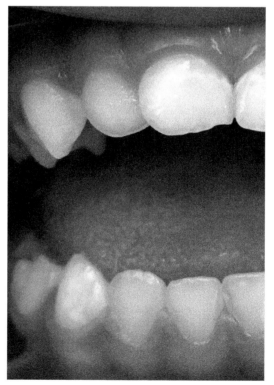

Fig. 1. White spot lesion.

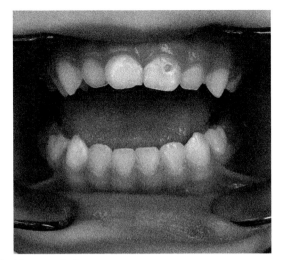

Fig. 2. Cavitated white spot lesion.

Streptococcus mutans is strongly associated with dental caries and has the ability to adhere to enamel. It is uniquely equipped to produce significant amounts of acid. Acids produced by bacterial fermentation of carbohydrates reduce the pH of dental plaque leading to demineralization of the enamel. Children are more likely to develop dental decay if *Mutans Streptococci* and *Lactobacillus* species are acquired at an early age.[17,18] Early acquisition of these bacterial strands often occur at a young age, as a result of horizontal or vertical bacterial transmission. Vertical transmission of bacteria often occurs through salivary spread from parent to child, whereas horizontal transmission occurs between other family members or friends to the child.[19]

ECC is a rapid form of tooth decay and was once called "baby bottle tooth decay" because the key cause of the disease is putting a child to bed with a bottle of milk or juice.[13,20,21] The American Academy of Pediatric Dentistry (AAPD) defines ECC as the presence of one or more decayed, noncavitated, or cavitated lesions and a missing or filled tooth surface due to caries in any primary tooth in a child under the age of 6 (**Fig. 3**).[20] ECC is often untreated in children under the age of 3 and is 5 times more

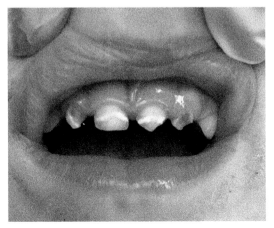

Fig. 3. Early childhood caries.

common than asthma.[14,22] Children who are given pacifying bottles of juice, milk, or formula to drink during the day or overnight are more likely to develop ECC.[13,20,21] Other factors that put children at risk for ECC include enamel defects, poor dental hygiene, a lack of fluoridated water, certain medications, mouth breathing, and frequent consumption of sugary snacks and drinks.[13,23,24]

Because of the aggressive nature of ECC, cavities can develop quickly, and if left untreated, can result in increased risk for severe dental infections. Untreated ECC may result in a medical emergency requiring hospitalization and emergent treatment. A dental infection is considered emergent when it presents as a facial cellulitis that approximates the submandibular or periorbital regions (**Fig. 4**). Hospital admission with intravenous antibiotics and consultation with a pediatric dentist is indicated at this stage.

THE ROLE OF THE PEDIATRICIAN IN ORAL HEALTH

Access to dental care is one of the barriers to improved oral health for children. This discrepancy is exacerbated by a shortage of pediatric dentists in the United States—especially ones who accept Medicaid.[14–16] Although the American Academy for Pediatrics (AAP) and the AAPD recommend that children visit a dentist every 6 months, beginning at 12 months of age, 22% of children under the age of 17 did not visit the dentist in the previous year.[25–27]

An intraoral examination and review of oral health care is a standard part of a well-child checkup. Preventive health services are delivered routinely by pediatricians and begin early in infancy on a regular, well-accepted schedule. Thus, pediatricians are ideal front-line providers who can detect oral health issues and begin the process of care and prevention at an early age. Pediatric health care professionals can provide counseling on caries prevention, caries risk assessment, and provision of a caries control treatment, such as fluoride varnish application.

Fluoride Varnish

The mechanism for fluoride administration is both topical and systemic. Fluoride reduces enamel dissolution and encourages enamel remineralization.[28] Fluoridated water is the least expensive and most effective way to deliver anti-caries benefits to communities.[29,30] Water fluoridation optimizes the level of fluoride in drinking water, which results in preeruptive and posteruptive protection of teeth.[31]

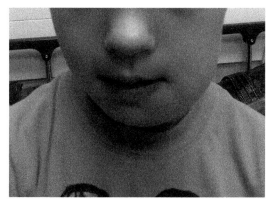

Fig. 4. Facial cellulitis.

Professionally applied topical fluorides (PATFs) are most effective at preventing caries when applied at regular intervals.[32] PATFs come in various forms, including gel, foam, rinses, and varnish. Fluoride varnishes are recommended for young children because they are less likely to be ingested in large quantities and adhere best to the tooth surface, increasing time of contact between the fluoride and tooth surface.[29,32] In the primary dentition, the effectiveness of varnish is 30% to 63.2%, and this is enhanced when combined with oral hygiene and dietary counseling.[33–35]

Before applying varnish, teeth should be dried with gauze to achieve maximum adherence to tooth structure. Parents and patients should be advised to avoid brushing for 6 hours after application, for maximum fluoride uptake. Fluoride application reduces decay by one-third and leads to significant cost savings in restorative dental care and associated hospital costs.[36,37] Most Medicaid programs reimburse for fluoride application.[37] All 50 states and the District of Columbia have Medicaid programs that reimburse medical providers for preventative dental care.[37]

In addition, self-administered fluorides, including dietary fluoride supplementation and fluoridated toothpaste, provide low fluoride concentrations.[38,39] Self-administered fluoride supplementation reduce caries by 32% to 72% in the primary dentition.[33] Need for dietary fluoride supplementation must be carefully evaluated and prescribed by a health care professional. Over-the-counter fluoridated toothpastes and mouth rinses reduce caries to a similar extent in children and adolescents.[40]

Health care providers must balance the benefits of caries prevention against the risk for development of enamel fluorosis. Enamel fluorosis is a form of hypomineralization and typically develops in children younger than 8 years of age before tooth maturation and emergence.[41] Caries susceptibility and sources of dietary fluoride should be considered before recommending fluoride therapies.[42–45]

Oral Health Risk Assessment

An oral health risk assessment should be administered periodically to all children. The AAPD has developed a caries risk-assessment tool for use by practitioners familiar with the clinical presentation of caries and factors related to caries initiation and progression.[46] Although radiographic assessment and microbiologic testing are included in the tool, they are not required. In addition, the AAP has developed the *Oral Health Risk Assessment Training for Pediatricians and Other Child Health Professionals*; this provides the elements of risk assessment and triage for infants and young children.[47] Risk should be reassessed periodically to account for changes in diet, oral hygiene, and general health conditions. Reassessment allows the practitioner to readdress and individualize preventive programs.

Anticipatory Guidance

Anticipatory guidance is the process of providing age-appropriate information to prepare parents for physical, emotional, and psychological milestones.[48] Anticipatory guidance specific to oral health emphasizes prevention of dental problems and should be integrated as part of comprehensive counseling during well-child visits. Anticipatory guidance and well-child visits reduce dental expenditures and decrease the number of hospitalizations among poor and near-poor children during the first 2 years of life.[49,50] The AAPD advocates oral health anticipatory guidance (**Table 1**).[25,51–53]

The cause of dental decay is trifold: oral hygiene, sugar consumption, and bacterial load. To reduce the risk of ECC, it is recommended that parents assist with twice daily brushing with the use of a fluoridated toothpaste, upon eruption of the first tooth. For children under the age of 3, a smear size amount of fluoridated toothpaste is indicated

Table 1 Anticipatory guidance	
Age	Recommendations
Birth to 6 mo	• Common oral findings of the newborn/infant: Gingival or palatal cyst of the newborn, Bohn nodule, cleft lip/palate, congenital epulis, neonatal teeth, ankyloglossia • Discourage napping or sleeping with the bottle • Encourage tooth brushing when first tooth erupts • Review teething patterns and palliative care
6–12 mo	• Encourage use of smear amount of fluoridated toothpaste • Evaluate need for in-office topical fluoride application • Refer to pediatric dentist to establish a dental home • Discuss mouth and tooth injury • Review teething patterns & palliative care • Discourage nonnutritive sucking on fingers and thumbs
12–36 mo	• Reinforce oral hygiene and diet modification • Evaluate need for in-office topical fluoride application • Reinforce oral injury prevention • Encourage discontinued use of bottle and pacifier • Evaluate early speech/language development
36+ mo	• Reinforce oral hygiene and diet modification • Transition to pea size of fluoridated toothpaste • Evaluate need for in-office topical fluoride application • Reinforce oral injury prevention • Encourage use of sports mouth guard • Evaluate speech/language development
Adolescence	• Reinforce oral hygiene and diet modification • Evaluate need for in-office topical fluoride application • Encourage use of sports mouth guard • Discuss oral health implications of intraoral piercings • Discuss drug and alcohol usage

(**Fig. 5**A), whereas a pea-sized amount of fluoridated toothpaste is indicated for children ages 3 to 6 (**Fig. 5**B).[54]

Parents should dispense the fluoridated toothpaste on a soft bristled brush that is age appropriate for the child. This task should be supervised to avoid excess fluoride intake and to ensure effective brushing. In addition, once teeth are in contact with one another, parents should incorporate flossing into the routine to prevent interproximal decay. Interproximal decay is common in children and can be detected on a dental radiograph (**Fig. 6**). If a child does not have an established dental home, interproximal decay can go undetected and over time will result in large, often nonrestorable decay.

Dietary choices affect oral health and the overall well-being of an individual. High-risk dietary habits are established by 12 months of age and are maintained throughout childhood.[55] In August of 2016, the American Heart Association released new guidelines indicating that children should consume less than 25 g (ie, 5 tablespoons) of added sugars daily. The guideline also recommends that children under the age of 2 should not consume foods or beverages with added sugars.[56] Children should not consume more than 4 to 6 ounces of juice per day. Juice should come from a cup, rather than a bottle or sippy cup, and should be paired with mealtime.[57]

In addition to juice and sugary snacks, one must also consider the frequency of milk consumption. One cup of 2% milk contains 12.5 g of sugar. Although milk contains many vitamins critical for growth and development, children who consume milk

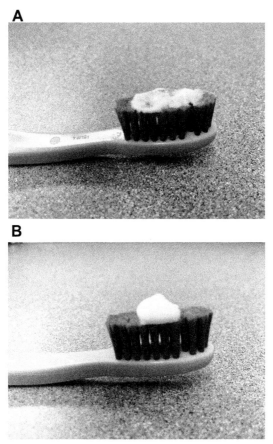

Fig. 5. Appropriate fluoridated toothpaste amounts for children. (*A*) Smear: under 3 years. (*B*) Pea sized: 3 to 6 years.

frequently throughout the day are at an increased risk for dental decay. In addition, sticky snacks and sweets should be avoided to reduce pit and fissure decay in posterior teeth (**Fig. 7**). Pit and fissure caries accounts for 80% to 90% of caries in permanent posterior teeth and 44% in primary posterior teeth.[58]

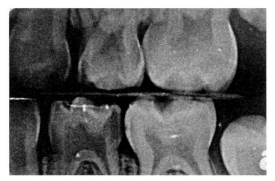

Fig. 6. Interproximal decay on a radiograph.

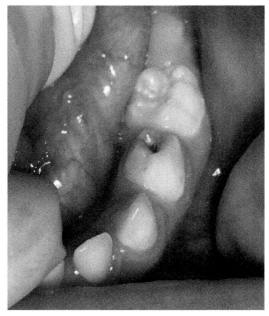

Fig. 7. Pit and fissure caries.

Interprofessional Collaboration

The concept of the dental home is based on the medical home model and is intended to improve access to oral care. A dental home is the ongoing relationship between the dentist and patient. It is inclusive of all aspects of oral health care that is delivered in a comprehensive, continuously accessible, family-centered way.[59]

Although the ideal setting for administration of oral health care is the dental home, when unavailable, pediatric health care providers should administer risk-based preventive oral health measures until a dental home is established. Creating collaborative relationships between physicians, physician assistants, nurse practitioners, and dentists is essential for increasing access to dental care for children while improving oral

---

Box 1
Anticipatory guidance

1. Infant oral hygiene instruction: Teeth should be brushed at least twice daily with caregiver supervision and assistance for children. For children with elevated dental caries risk, consider using a pea-sized amount of toothpaste or an amount equivalent to the child's fifth-digit fingernail. Flossing should begin as soon as adjacent teeth are in contact and for surfaces at which 2 teeth touch and they can no longer be cleansed with a toothbrush.

2. Counseling regarding nonnutritive oral habits: Use of pacifiers in the first year of life may prevent sudden infant death syndrome.[56] Sucking habits (eg, pacifiers or digits) of sufficient frequency, duration, and intensity may be associated with dentoalveolar deformations. Some changes persist past cessation of the habit. Professional evaluation is indicated for nonnutritive sucking habits that continue beyond 3 years of age.[53]

3. Age-appropriate information regarding dental injury prevention: Parents should cover sharp corners of household furnishings at the level of walking toddlers, ensure use of car safety seats, and be aware of electrical cord risk for mouth injury. Properly fitted mouth guards are indicated for youths involved in sporting activities that carry a risk of orofacial injury.

and overall health. Establishment of these relationships allows for comprehensive care and collaborative efforts during dental emergencies.

In today's health care environment, working interprofessionally to provide patient-centered medicine is the norm. Pediatricians are used to working with and making referrals to other health care providers. Pediatrician s' referral rates to pediatric dentists for children with oral disease or with elevated risk for caries are low however.[60] Several factors explain the low dental referral rates in children.[60,61] Having a better understanding of common dental diseases and emergencies that require referral to a dentist will help improve referral rates (**Box 1**, **Table 2**). Often, the first step of timely establishment of a dental home is a referral from the physician.

Table 2
Common pediatric dental emergencies

Condition	Description	Treatment
Toothache	Common causes: Trauma Dental decay Erupting wisdom teeth in adolescence	Analgesics for discomfort Evaluate need for antibiotics if dental abscess or facial cellulitis are present Refer to dentist for treatment
Dental concussion	Often the result of a hit to a tooth, without increased mobility or displacement. Often associated with pain upon biting or palpation of tooth	Analgesics for discomfort Soft diet for 2–3 d Often heals without further complications
Dental luxation	Displacement of the tooth from the socket in any other direction, besides axially. Often associated with alveolar bone fracture and tooth mobility	Analgesics for discomfort Soft diet for 2–3 d *Urgent referral* to dentist for further clinical and radiographic evaluation and possible treatment
Dental intrusion/ extrusion	Displacement of the tooth in axial direction. May be pushed into the socket (intrusion) or displaced out of the socket (extrusion)	Analgesics for discomfort Soft diet for 2–3 d *Urgent referral* to dentist for further clinical and radiographic evaluation and possible treatment
Dental avulsion	Complete displacement of the entire tooth from the socket	Analgesics for discomfort Primary tooth: No treatment necessary, reimplantation of the tooth is not indicated Permanent tooth: *Emergent referral* to dentist. Immediate reimplantation and splint placement necessary to stabilize tooth
Tooth fracture	Fracture of the coronal portion of the tooth. Varies in severity depending on depth of fracture	Analgesics for discomfort Soft diet until treated by dentist *Urgent referral* to dentist
Tongue or lip laceration	Laceration of the soft tissue of the lip or tongue. May be superficial laceration or through and through laceration	Evaluate depth and extent of laceration Evaluate need for immediate suture placement Analgesics for discomfort

Data from Copenhagen University Hospital and the International Association of Dental Traumatology. Dental Trauma Guide. Available at: https://dentaltraumaguide.org/dtg-members-frontpage/. Accessed May 1, 2017.

Ideally, pediatric health care providers should refer children to a pediatric dentist. This is especially important for a child that presents with ECC because pediatric dentists are able to provide sedation and surgical treatment options for young children. The AAPD Web site provides a list of pediatric dentists within the community. If there is not a pediatric dentist within close proximity, a general dentist can help manage immediate dental needs.

Pediatricians may also need to refer to an oral surgeon to help further evaluate oral pathology lesions. Oral surgeons are an excellent resource for oral pathology excisions and biopsies for both children and adults. Other specialists within the dental community include periodontists, endodontists, orthodontists, and prosthodontists. It is uncommon for medical providers to make a direct referral to these other dental specialists.

The relationship among medical and dental health care providers should be symbiotic. Dental professionals often refer back to medical providers for consultations before sedation for dental work or for medical workup based on clinical extraoral or intraoral findings. Working interprofessionally within the medical community is critical for providing comprehensive, patient-centered care to children today.

REFERENCES

1. Centers for Disease Control and Prevention. Oral health data. 2016. Available at: https://www.cdc.gov/oralhealth/basics/childrens-oral-health/index.html. Accessed May 5, 2017.
2. Dye BA, Xianfen L, Beltrán-Aguilar ED. Selected oral health indicators in the United States 2005–2008. NCHS Data Brief, no. 96. Hyattsville (MD): National Center for Health Statistics, Centers for Disease Control and Prevention; 2012.
3. Byck GR, Cooksey JA, Russinof H. Safety-net dental clinics. J Am Dent Assoc 2005;136(7):1013–21.
4. Edelstein BL. Disparities in oral health and access to care: findings of national surveys. Ambul Pediatr 2002;2(2):141–7.
5. Gift HC, Reisine ST, Larach DC. The social impact of dental problems and visits. Am J Public Health 1992;82(12):1663–8.
6. Seirawan H, Faust S, Mulligan R. The impact of oral health on the academic performance of disadvantaged children. Am J Public Health 2012;102(9):1729–34.
7. Acs G, Lodolini G, Kaminsky S, et al. Effect of nursing caries on body weight in a pediatric population. Pediatr Dent 1992;14(5):302–5.
8. Nyaradi A, Li J, Hickling S, et al. The role of nutrition in children's neurocognitive development, from pregnancy through childhood. Front Hum Neurosci 2013;7:97.
9. Blumenshine SL, Vann WF, Gizlice Z, et al. Children's school performance: impact of general and oral health. J Public Health Dent 2008;68(2):82–7.
10. de Paula DF, Santos NC, daSilva ET, et al. Pyschosocial impact of dental esthetics on quality of life in adolescents. Angle Orthod 2009;79(6):1188–93.
11. Zhang M, McGrath C, Hägg U. Impact of malocclusion and its treatment on quality of life: A literature review. Int J Paediatr Dent 2006;16(6):381–7.
12. White BA, Caplan DJ, Weintraub JA. A quarter century of changes in oral health in the United States. J Dent Educ 1995;59(1):19–57.
13. US Department of Health and Human Services and the National Institute of Dental and Craniofacial Research. Oral health in America: a report of the surgeon general. Rockville (MD): US Department of Health and Human Services, National Institute of Dental and Craniofacial Research, National Institutes of Health; 2000.
14. Vargas CM, Ronzio CR. Disparities in early childhood caries. BMC Oral Health 2006;6(Suppl 1):S3.

15. U.S. Department of Health and Human Services. A national call to action to promote oral health. NIH Publication No. 03–5303. Rockville (MD): U.S. Department of Health and Human Services, Public Health Service, Centers for Disease Control and Prevention, and the National Institutes of Health, National Institute of Dental and Craniofacial Research; 2003. Available at: https://www.nidcr.nih.gov/DataStatistics/SurgeonGeneral/NationalCalltoAction/Documents/NationalCallToAction.pdf. Accessed May 5, 2017.

16. Bloom B, Cohen RA, Freeman G. Summary health statistics for U.S. children: National Health Interview Survey, 2008. National Center for Health Statistics. Vital Health Stat 10 2009;(244):1–81. Available at: https://www.cdc.gov/nchs/data/series/sr_10/sr10_244.pdf. Accessed May 5, 2017.

17. Harris R, Nicoll AD, Adair PM, et al. Risk factors for dental caries in young children: A systematic review of the literature. Community Dent Health 2004;21(suppl 1):71–85.

18. Kanasi E, Johansson J, Lu SC, et al. Microbial risk markers for childhood caries in pediatrician's offices. J Dent Res 2010;89(4):378–83.

19. Berkowitz RJ. Mutans streptococci: acquisition and transmission. Pediatr Dent 2006;28(2):106–9.

20. American Academy of Pediatric Dentistry, Counsel on Clinical Affairs. Policy on early childhood caries (ACC): classifications, consequences, and preventive strategies. Oral Health Policies Reference Manual 2014;37(6):50–2.

21. American Academy of Pediatric Dentistry. The state of little teeth. Available at: http://www.aapd.org/assets/1/7/State_of_Little_Teeth_Final.pdf. Accessed May 5, 2017.

22. Tinanoff N, Reisine S. Update on early childhood caries since the Surgeon General's Report. Acad Pediatr 2009;9(6):396–403.

23. Davies GN. Early childhood caries: a synopsis. Community Dent Oral Epidemiol 1998;26(suppl):106–16.

24. Seow WK. Biological mechanisms of early childhood caries. Community Dent Oral Epidemiol 1998;26(suppl):8–27.

25. American Academy of Pediatric Dentistry. Guideline on periodicity of examination, preventive dental services, anticipatory guidance, and oral treatment for children. Pediatr Dent 2005;27(7 suppl):84–6.

26. Hale KJ. Oral health risk assessment timing and establishment of the dental home. Pediatrics 2003;111(5 Pt):1113–6.

27. Bell JF, Huebner CE, Reed SC. Oral health need and access to dental services: evidence from the National Survey of Children's Health, 2007. Matern Child Health J 2012;16(suppl 1):S27–34.

28. Cate JM, Featherstone JD. Mechanistic aspects of the interactions between fluoride and dental enamel. Crit Rev Oral Biol Med 1991;2(3):283–96.

29. Centers for Disease Control and Prevention. Recommendations for using fluoride to prevent and control dental caries in the United States. MMWR Recomm Rep 2001;50(RR-14):1–42.

30. Griffin SO, Jones K, Tomar SL. An economic evaluation of community water fluoridation. J Public Health Dent 2001;61(2):78–86.

31. Singh KA, Spencer AJ. Relative effects of pre- and post-eruption water fluoride on caries experience by surface type of permanent first molars. Community Dent Oral Epidemiol 2004;32(6):435–6.

32. Hawkins R, Locker D, Nobel J, et al. Prevention. Part 7: professionally applied topical fluorides for caries prevention. Br Dent J 2003;195(6):313–7.

33. Bader JD, Rozier GR, Lohr KN, et al. Physicians' roles in preventing dental caries in preschool children: a summary of the evidence for the U.S. Preventive Services Task Force. Am J Prev Med 2004;26(4):315–25.

34. Marinho VC, Higgins JP, Logan S, et al. Fluoride varnishes for preventing dental caries in children and adolescents. Cochrane Database Syst Rev 2002;(3):CD002279.

35. Weintraub JA, Ramos-Gomez F, Jue B, et al. Fluoride varnish efficacy in preventing early childhood caries. J Dent Res 2006;85(2):172–6.

36. Helfenstein U, Steiner M. Fluoride varnishes (Duraphat): a meta-analysis. Community Dent Oral Epidemiol 1994;22:1–5.

37. The Pew Charitable Trust. Reimbursing physicians for fluoride varnish. August 29, 2011. Available at: http://www.pewtrusts.org/en/research-and-analysis/analysis/2011/08/29/reimbursing-physicians-for-fluoride-varnish. Accessed May 5, 2017.

38. Lynch RJ, Navada R, Walia R. Low-levels of fluoride in plaque and saliva and their effects on demineralisation and remineralisation of enamel: role of fluoride toothpastes. Int Dent J 2004;54(5 suppl 1):304–9.

39. Marinho VC, Higgins JP, Logan S, et al. Topical fluoride (toothpastes, mouthrinses, gels or varnishes) for preventing dental caries in children and adolescents. Cochrane Database Syst Rev 2003;(4):CD002782.

40. Marinho VC, Higgins JP, Sheiham A, et al. One topical fluoride (toothpastes, mouthrinses, gels, or varnishes) versus another for preventing dental caries in children and adolescents. Cochrane Database Syst Rev 2004;(1):CD002780.

41. Pang DT, Vann WF. The use of fluoride-containing toothpastes in young children: the scientific evidence for recommending a small quantity. Pediatr Dent 1992; 14(6):384–7.

42. Featherstone JD. The caries balance: the basis for caries management by risk assessment. Oral Health Prev Dent 2004;2(suppl 1):259–64.

43. Jacobsen P, Young D. The use of topical fluoride to prevent or reverse dental caries. Spec Care Dentist 2003;23(5):177–9.

44. Warren JJ, Levy SM. Systemic fluoride: sources, amounts, and effects of ingestion. Dent Clin North Am 1999;43(4):695–711.

45. Levy SM, Kohout FJ, Kiritsy MC, et al. Infant's fluoride ingestion from water, supplements and dentifrice. J Am Dent Assoc 1995;126(12):1625–32.

46. American Academy of Pediatric Dentistry Council on Clinical Affairs. Policy on use of a caries-risk assessment tool (CAT) for infants, children, and adolescents. Pediatr Dent 2005–2006;27(7 suppl):25–7. Available at. www.aapd.org/media/Policies_Guidelines/P_CariesRiskAssess.pdf. Accessed May 5, 2017.

47. American Academy of Pediatrics. Oral health risk assessment training for pediatricians and other child health professionals. Elk Grove Village (IL): American Academy of Pediatrics; 2005.

48. Lewis CW, Boulter S, Keels MA, et al. Oral health and pediatricians: results of a national survey. Acad Pediatr 2009;9(6):457–61.

49. Hakim RB, Bye BV. Effectiveness of compliance with pediatric preventive care guidelines among Medicaid beneficiaries. Pediatrics 2001;108(1):90–7.

50. Savage MR, Lee JY, Kotch JB, et al. Early preventive dental visits: effects on subsequent utilization and costs. Pediatrics 2004;114(4):e418–23. Available at: www.pediatrics.org/cgi/content/full/114/4/e418. Accessed May 5, 2017.

51. Nowak AJ, Casamassimo PS. Using anticipatory guidance to provide early dental intervention. J Am Dent Assoc 1995;126(8):1156–63.

52. Nowak AJ, Warren JJ. Infant oral health and oral habits. Pediatr Clin North Am 2000;47(5):1043–66.

53. American Academy of Pediatrics, Bright Futures Steering Committee. Bright futures: guidelines for health supervision of infants, children, and adolescents. In: Hagen JF, Shaw JS, Duncan PM, editors. 4th edition. Elk Grove Village (IL): American Academy of Pediatrics; 2008.

54. Wright JT, Hanson N, Ristic H, et al. Fluoride toothpaste efficacy and safety in children younger than 6 years. J Am Dent Assoc 2014;145(2):182–9.

55. Douglass JM. Response to Tinano and Palmer: dietary determinants of dental caries and dietary recommendations for preschool children. J Public Health Dent 2000;60(3):207–9.

56. American Heart Association. AHA guideline on sugar consumption 2016. Available at: http://newsroom.heart.org/news/children-should-eat-less-than-25-grams-of-added-sugars-daily. Accessed May 5, 2017.

57. American Academy of Pediatrics Committee on Nutrition. Policy statement: the use and misuse of fruit juices in pediatrics. Pediatrics 2001;107(5):1210–3.

58. Beauchamp J, Caufield PW, Crall JJ, et al. Evidence-based clinical recommendations for the use of pit-and-fissure sealants: a report of the American Dental Association Council on Scientific Affairs. J Am Dent Assoc 2008;139(3):257–68.

59. Section on Pediatric Dentistry and Oral Health. Preventive oral health intervention for pediatricians. Pediatrics 2008;122(6):1387–94. Available at: http://pediatrics.aappublications.org/content/pediatrics/122/6/1387.full.pdf. Accessed May 5, 2017.

60. Long CM, Quiñonez RB, Beil HA, et al. Pediatricians' assessments of caries risk and need for a dental evaluation in preschool aged children. BMC Pediatr 2012; 12:49.

61. dela Cruz GG, Rozier RG, Slade GD. Dental screening and referral of young children by pediatric primary care providers. Pediatrics 2004;114:e642–52.

Otitis Media
Beyond the Examining Room

Deborah R. Welling, AuD, CCC/A, FAAA[a],*, Carol A. Ukstins, MS, CCC/A, FAAA[b]

KEYWORDS

- Conductive hearing loss • IDEA Part C • Medical model • Mixed hearing loss
- Educational model • Chronic Otitis media • Sensorineural hearing loss
- Special education

KEY POINTS

- The stages of otitis media are connected with various degrees and types of hearing loss.
- Hearing loss secondary to otitis media can have far-reaching effects on receptive and expressive language development.
- A collaborative approach to early intervention can significantly improve treatment outcomes.
- The educational impact of hearing loss on school-aged children includes auditory deprivation, psychosocial implications, and overall academic success.
- The team of professionals available to assist medical providers in the management of sequelae of otitis media includes clinical audiologists, educational audiologists, speech-language pathologists, and skilled professionals in the educational setting.

INTRODUCTION

According to the 2016 guidelines codeveloped by the American Academy of Otolaryngology–Head and Neck Surgery Foundation (AAO-HNSF), the American Academy of Pediatrics (AAP), and the American Academy of Family Physicians (AAFP),[1] otitis media with effusion (OME) is a term used to describe the presence of fluid in the middle ear without signs or symptoms of acute infection, whereas acute otitis media (OM) indicates the rapid onset of signs and symptoms associated with inflammation, often including pain and a bulging eardrum. Numerous additional terms further define and describe the condition. For example, the time course of the disease may be chronic or acute, and the effusion may vary from serous (thin) to purulent (puslike), or a combination.[2] The focus of this article is not to address the varying forms and stages of OM nor the associated medical treatments. This article discusses the concomitant hearing loss and its resulting nonmedical impact.

Disclosure: There are no commercial or financial conflicts of interest for either author.
[a] Department of Speech-Language Pathology, Seton Hall University, 400 South Orange Avenue, South Orange, NJ 07079, USA; [b] Newark Public Schools, Office of Special Education, 2 Cedar Street, Newark, NJ 07102, USA
* Corresponding author.
E-mail address: Deborah.welling@shu.edu

Although the specific prevalence and incidence data depend on the specific source and population they reference, OM is extremely common, particularly in the pediatric population. In the same 2016 clinical practice guidelines, OME is described as an occupational hazard of childhood, with about 90% of children experiencing OME before school age.[1] In addition, according to the AAP, OM is the most common condition for which antibacterial agents are prescribed.[3] Clearly, medical management of this condition is critically important.

However, OM and its concomitant hearing loss further affect other areas, such as speech-language development, academic achievement, and psychosocial skills. Moreover, a review of the abundant literature on this topic shows not only the variety of developmental and functional areas potentially affected but also the extreme variability in severity and the temporary or permanent nature of the condition. Therefore, there can be no one-size-fits-all intervention strategy and a collaborative effort among professionals (physician, audiologist, speech-language pathologist, teacher, and others) will be essential if clinicians are to achieve best outcomes for patients.

Connecting Disorder to Sensory Deprivation

Middle ear disorder requires a unique focus of treatment in its varying stages, and hearing loss is the most common complication.[4] Therefore, the view of OM cannot be a single continuum of disorder-treatment-resolution but must be one of addressing the impact that the resulting hearing loss will have on the patient's activities of daily living. Speech and language development, academic achievement, psychosocial impact and overall communication abilities must be considered as part of the treatment plan. The authors therefore revise the model from disorder-treatment-resolution to disorder-treatment-rehabilitation-educational/vocational planning-resolution–continuation of follow-up services and monitoring. It is encouraging to note that this multidisciplinary collaborative perspective is also reflected in the 2016 codeveloped practice guidelines.[1]

Hearing loss associated with OM can vary from slight/minimal to moderately severe, can be unilateral or bilateral, is predominantly conductive (conductive hearing loss), and the severity of the disorder has been found to correspond significantly with the severity of the resulting hearing loss.[5] Notwithstanding, patients with preexisting sensorineural hearing loss can also have middle ear disorders resulting in a mixed hearing loss of both sensorineural and conductive components. Although less commonly highlighted, there is the risk for developing sensorineural hearing loss as a complication of the chronic form of the disease.[6-8] It is therefore imperative to actively treat pediatric patients diagnosed with chronic OM, with the aim of preventing this from occurring.[6]

Regardless of the type and degree of the resulting hearing loss (**Table 1**), the periods of sensory deprivation do not always fit into stereotypical scenarios. With regard to hearing loss of minimal degree (16–25 decibels hearing level [dB HL]), evidence exists indicating that although some individuals may appear to have no observable speech-language or academic difficulties, others experience considerable difficulties. In addition, even though children with minimal hearing loss may appear to catch up in some areas, difficulties in select domains continue into adulthood.[9] In cases in which the resulting sensory deficit is more severe, the manifestation of hearing loss can take on many different forms, seemingly varying from child to child. It is important therefore to understand that these periods of auditory deprivation, slight to severe, and temporary to permanent, have negative consequences on speech and language development and the like.

Hearing loss secondary to OM has been documented as a risk factor for auditory processing difficulties[10-12] as well as having an impact on educational access and achievement, and psychosocial development. Nevertheless, the behavioral symptoms are subjective and usually ignored by teachers and parents.[13] Studies have shown that parental concern for their children's hearing has low sensitivity and very low positive predictive value for detecting hearing loss, particularly with slight and mild degrees.[14,15] A study that investigated parental perception of hearing loss as a secondary characteristic of OME found that less than 19.7% of parents were cognizant of the presence of hearing loss in their children. This finding crossed socioeconomic boundaries and educational achievement levels of the parents. The referenced article stated that, if parental suspicion had been relied on as the first screening, at least 80% of the OME cases would have been missed and concluded that parental suspicion is inadequate for identification of mild hearing loss as caused by OME.[16]

Table 1
Types of hearing loss

Type of Hearing Loss	Typical Audiometric Findings	Characteristics	Common Causes
Conductive	• Air conduction outside of normal range • Bone conduction within normal range • Significant air/bone gaps • Speech discrimination scores very good to excellent • Tympanograms abnormal; eg, B, C, As, or Ad, depending on specific cause • Otoacoustic emissions (all types) absent because of the conductive disorder	• Unilateral or bilateral • Temporary or permanent • Fluctuations of loudness common depending on the cause • Discrimination of the speech signal is generally intact when speech is made loud enough • Loss of sensitivity without the distortional aspect that accompanied sensorineural hearing loss • May be accompanied by ringing, buzzing, or dizziness • Frequently medically and/or surgically treatable	• Impacted cerumen • Otitis media • Perforated tympanic membrane • Ossicular discontinuity • Otosclerosis

Conductive Audiogram
A moderate conductive heaing loss

(continued on next page)

Table 1
(continued)

Type of Hearing Loss	Typical Audiometric Findings	Characteristics	Common Causes
Sensorineural	• Air conduction outside of normal range • Bone conduction outside of normal range • No air/bone gaps; ie, air and bone conduction thresholds are equally abnormal • Speech discrimination is impaired to varying degrees, especially in background noise • Tympanograms typically normal (type A) because disorder is not in the conductive mechanism • Otoacoustic emission may be present for lesser degrees of hearing loss	• Unilateral or bilateral • Generally permanent condition • Loss of sensitivity likely to include distortional aspects • Discrimination of the speech signal is impaired to varying degrees • Fluctuation in speech discrimination ability is also common • Additional difficulty with understanding speech in noisy environments • May be accompanied by tinnitus and/or dizziness • Generally not medically or surgically treatable	• Congenital and/or genetic • Perinatal causes; eg, anoxia, CHARGE, • Diseases and infections • Noise exposure • Ototoxicity • Presbycusis

Sensorineural Audiogram
A mild sloping to severe sensorineural hearing loss

(continued on next page)

Table 1
(continued)

Type of Hearing Loss	Typical Audiometric Findings	Characteristics	Common Causes
Mixed	• Air conduction thresholds outside of normal range • Bone conduction thresholds outside of normal range • Air/bone gaps are present; ie, both air and bone responses are impaired, but air conduction thresholds are more abnormal than bone • Tympanograms are likely abnormal; this depends on the specific causes creating the conductive and sensorineural components • Otoacoustic emissions are most likely absent because of the presence of the conductive component of the hearing loss	• Unilateral or bilateral • Fluctuations in loudness possible depending on the particular causes involved • Discrimination of the speech signal is impaired to varying degrees, depending on the causes • Additional difficulty with understanding speech in noisy environments • May be accompanied by tinnitus and/or dizziness • Sensorineural component is generally not medically or surgically treatable • Conductive portion of the hearing loss may be medically and/or surgically treatable, depending on the cause	• Any combination of conductive and sensorineural conditions; eg, otitis media in a child with preexisting congenital hearing loss • Craniofacial abnormalities

Mixed Audiogram
A moderate to severe mixed hearing loss

Reproduced with permission from Deborah R. Welling and Carol A. Ukstins.

Inasmuch as hearing loss can be missed as a diagnostic precept, there are many reported commonly observed behaviors associated with OME and its concomitant hearing loss (**Box 1**). It is the identification of these behaviors that serve as red flags to medical providers that further interventions are warranted, and the point at which

Box 1
Common behaviors and symptoms that indicate hearing loss

Some of the most common behaviors observed for individuals with hearing loss.

Symptoms common to infants and very young children with hearing loss

- Child does not awaken or stir in response to loud sounds
- Child responds well visually but does not turn in response to sound
- Child does not respond to own name
- Child's babbling diminishes or changes in quality/character
- Child's first words do not emerge as expected at approximately 12 months of age
- Child's utterances are hard to understand
- Child speaks inappropriately loud or soft
- With unilateral hearing loss child may consistently respond to 1 side only
- Child may have a habit of pointing to things instead of asking

Symptoms common in hearing loss secondary to middle ear disorder

- Inconsistent responses to sound
- Frequently say "What?" or "Huh?"
- Volume of voice may be inappropriately soft
- Apparent difficulty hearing, understanding, and responding
- Pulling or tugging on the ear
- Irritability
- Sleep disturbances
- Ear pain
- Drainage from the ear
- Fever
- Congestion
- Decreased appetite

Symptoms of hearing loss of various types

- Inconsistent responses to sound
- Apparent difficulty hearing
- Volume of voice inappropriately loud or soft
- Poor speech intelligibility
- Confusions with similar-sounding words
- Lack of or inappropriate response during conversation
- Frequently saying "What, huh?" or asking for repetition
- Listens to television, radio, and so forth at louder than normal volumes
- Difficulty understanding in crowded settings
- Difficulty understanding when multiple speakers are present
- Difficulty hearing and understanding when a speaker's face is not visible
- Additional difficulty hearing and understanding in noisy settings

Symptoms of psychosocial impact of hearing loss

- Displays embarrassment when responding inappropriately in conversation
- Isolates and withdraws from social situations
- Displays feelings of stress, anxiety, and depression
- Fatigues more easily
- Displays frustration and annoyance when experiencing conversational difficulty
- May display irritability, negativism, and anger

Symptoms of children with hearing loss in a classroom

- Distracted by background noise
- Difficulty with speech and language
- Difficulty discriminating words that sound alike
- Difficulty hearing and following directions
- Frequent need for repetition or clarification of directions and important information
- Difficulty locating the sound source if it is not in the line of vision
- Inability to attend to stories read aloud
- Use of gestures instead of verbal expressions
- Pointing to things instead of asking
- Poor vocabulary
- Inconsistent behavior from day to day
- Inappropriate responses to questions or comments
- Difficulty following rapid conversational exchanges
- Behaviors of inattention may be confused with or misdiagnosed as attention-deficit disorder/attention-deficit/hyperactivity disorder

Reproduced with permission from Deborah R. Welling and Carol A. Ukstins.

professional collaboration begins. Regardless of age, successful intervention outcomes rely on the timely identification and referral for additional services.[17] In referencing **Box 1**, medical providers may find it useful to rephrase 1 or more of the noted behaviors into the form of a question to the parent or primary caretaker; for example, "Does your child listen to the television at a louder than normal volume?" The answers provided may reveal valuable case history information when identifying the presence of hearing loss concomitant to OME.

Birth Through 36 Months (the Early Intervention Years)

During the earliest stages of life, the schedule of routine medical visits related to well-child checks and immunizations lends itself to the timely identification of illnesses and disorders. Many new parents are also more likely to schedule medical visits at the first signs of abnormal behaviors suggesting that the infant may be developing an illness. During this stage of life, the middle ear structures relative to the shape and size of the other craniofacial structures make children of this age range more susceptible to otitis media in its various forms.[1] Throughout this crucial language-learning period, even slight decreases in auditory sensitivity secondary to OM can have far-reaching impacts on the skills necessary for normal speech, language, and literacy development, and later auditory and language processing as well.[11,18–20]

Table 2
Auditory-verbal development in typically developing children with normal hearing.

Ages (mo)	Input: Auditory Development	Output: Speech Production/Spoken Language

Birth to 3	Reactions to sounds:
	  Startle reflex, eye blink/eye widening, cessation of activity, limb movement, head turn toward or away, grimacing/crying, sucking, arousal, breathing change
	Speech perception abilities:
	• Can identify individual phonemes
	• Capable of detecting virtually every phoneme
	• Prefers vowels
	Prosody/suprasegmentals:
	• Prefers human voice
	• Attentive to the rise and fall on intonation pattern
	• Attends to patterns of speech
	• Prefers native language to all others
	Identification:
	• Identifies mother's voice
	• Prefers songs heard prenatally
		Reflexive
		  Coos, gurgles, reflexive sounds
		Physical response to sounds:
		  Stilling, rhythmic movement, searching for sounds source
		Vocalization:
		  Goo sounds, laughter
		  Quasi resonant nuclei, immature vowel-like sounds

3–4	Prosody/suprasegmentals: • Prefers utterances with intonation variation vs flat voice • Discriminates high and low sounds	
4–7	Early auditory feedback: Auditory tuning in: • Listening to language for longer periods of time • Shows awareness of environmental sounds • Can be behaviorally pacified by music or song Speech perception • Recognition of mother's voice • Reacts to vocal mood differences Localization: • Localization to sound begins to emerge from eye gaze to head turn to localization to specific sound sources (directly related to motor development) Auditory memory: • Beginning of auditory memory (distinguishes between voices of familiar people vs strangers)	Expanding vocal repertoire: vocal play FRN, vowel-like sounds, consonantlike sounds, CV and VC syllables emerge Play with streams of sounds, intonational patterns, raspberries, squeals, loudness play Vocal turn-taking exchanges with parent
5	Early auditory comprehension: • Responds to own name Suprasegmentals/prosody: • Discriminates own language from others with same prosody	Vocalization: • CV syllable and some VC syllable vocalizations • Imitates pitch tone

(continued on next page)

Table 2
(continued)

Ages (mo)	Input: Auditory Development	Output: Speech Production/Spoken Language
6	Correlation between achievements and speech perception and later word understanding, word production, and phrase production Speech perception: • Preference for vowel ends Early auditory feedback: Listens to self in vocal play Auditory identification: • Begins to recognize own name and the names of family members Reliable localization: • Begins to respond to directives Selective auditory attention: • Diverts attention from one activity to a more desirable activity based on auditory input The sound with meaning connection: The melody is the message. Child interprets parents' intention by listening and reacting to tone of voice change. Happens before word comprehension	Vocalization: • May produce recognizable vowels:/u/a/i/
8–10	Synaptogenesis: Explosion of synaptic growth may be related to change in perception and production Phonotactic regularities and prosody: Sensitive to regularities in word boundaries in infant-directed speech even in another language Begins storing sound patterns for words, although no meaning yet Auditory comprehension: Begins to comprehend words	Vocalization: canonical babble • Achieves strings of reduplicated and alternated syllable production; timing of syllable production sounds speechlike, stress patterns • Vowels, consonants becoming distinct Increased vocal turn-taking: Once true babble attained, parents expect more speechlike utterances Primitive speech acts Expressing intentions nonverbally
8–14		Protowords: Words invented by child not adult, but have consistent meaning. Such as "la-la" for blanket
9	Speech perception: Prefers nonwords composed of high phonotactic components Auditory attention: Sustained auditory attention: Attends to auditory-based activities for increased periods of time Phonotactic probabilities Predicting likelihood of certain sound sequences, listening preference for nonwords with high phonotactic probability vs those with low probability	Intentionality: "I know what I mean" • Child attains cognitive/communication intents • Achieves means-end concept • Uses vocal/verbal means to achieve ends in combination with visual and gestural mechanisms Vocalization: • Variegated babble: adjacent and following syllables are not identical

(continued on next page)

Table 2
(continued)

Ages (mo)	Input: Auditory Development	Output: Speech Production/Spoken Language
9–12		9–12 mo: speech to communicate • Sound imitation of common household items and animals • Distinct word approximations and in some cases early single-word utterances take place of crying to fulfill wants and needs • Verbal nicknames for distinct object and people develop and remain consistent for that object or person
10	Auditory tuning in: Narrows auditory attention and speech perception: tunes in to mother language, loses universal interest in all speech sounds	
10–16		Phonetically consistent forms Speech sounds that have sound-meaning relationships, such as "puda" for the family cat First words: context bound Following the first word, during the next few months, children add an average of 8–11 words to their vocabularies each month
11	Speech perception: Identifies allophones and word boundaries	Variegated babble Word approximations
12	Speech perception: Hears word and consonant boundaries	

	Ages 12–24 mo: Exploring and Expanding	
Ages (mo)	Listening: Auditory Comprehension	Speech Production and Spoken Language
12–18	Early auditory comprehension: Odd mappings of words Child attends to whole sentence Is able to follow commands Fully aware of the names for familiar objects and family members Auditory environment: Derives obvious pleasure from auditory activities like music, playing with friends, laughing, and being read to Auditory experience: Listening to speech for long periods of time is essential to the ultimate use of even single words	Overextension and underextension of words Language develops as a direct correlation of using that developing speech to ultimately gain a desired outcome through a communication interaction between the speaker and the listener Gradual decontextualization (to 18 mo) Says first clear distinct word and assigns that word to a single distinct object or person

(continued on next page)

Table 2 (continued)		
Ages 12–24 mo: Exploring and Expanding		
Ages (mo)	**Listening: Auditory Comprehension**	**Speech Production and Spoken Language**
16–20		Fast mapping: Ability to learn words in 1 or few exposures
18	Auditory vocabulary Tremendous growth in vocabulary comprehension, 100–200 words understood	First 50 words used: a first language Growth in expressive ability, tremendous growth in 1 word usage
18–24	Auditory localization: Independently seeks out a sound source in another room Auditory comprehension Understands and follows verbal directions with 2 critical elements Begins to respond appropriately to "What?" and "Where?" questions	Word spurt: vocabulary spurt Naming theory seems to be a bias for noun usage, naming people, objects; occurs for most children when they hit first 50-word mark Begins to sing along with songs or mimic the rhythm of a nursery rhyme
Ages 2–3 y		
Age (mo)	**Listening**	**Speaking**
24–36	Auditory identification: Identifies a sound and shares that identification with another person with exuberance. Desires to share auditory information with another person Auditory memory: Shares auditory experiences from memory (left brain) Sings complete or nearly complete songs from memory (right brain)	Cognitive/semantic: Two-word semantic relations, and 3-word-plus utterances Spoken language and play: Holds a seemingly appropriate conversation with an inanimate object while playing Phonology Presyntactic period
26–32		Phoneme repetition Vocabulary size seems related to ability to repeat phoneme combinations, especially initial position in nonwords
By 36		Early syntactic: Recombination of 2-word plus 2-word utterances Early multiple word utterances, correct word order Early morphology: "ing"

Adapted from Perigoe CB, Paterson MM. Understanding auditory development and the child with hearing loss. In: Welling DR, Ukstins CA, editors. Fundamentals of audiology for the speech-language pathologist, 1st edition. Burlington: Jones and Bartlett; 2015; with permission.

The connection between early developing listening skills and speech and language development is well established.[21] **Table 2** presents a chart that highlights the auditory developmental milestones from birth to 36 months and the speech and language correlates of each of those skills.

Services available under the Individuals with Disabilities Education Act (IDEA) Part C (Early Intervention) may be in the form of speech and language therapy as well as audiological services to address the deleterious effects of OM on speech and language development. In the continuum of services, the eligibility for Part C is defined by the federal law but is determined through each state's guidelines. The federal law defines eligibility for Part C services based on (1) developmental delays in the areas of cognitive development, physical development including vision and hearing, communication development, and social or emotional development; or (2) a diagnosed physical or mental condition that has a high probability of resulting in developmental delay.[22] The term developmental delay is defined by each state.[23]

Although direct services for hearing loss in IDEA Part C speak to permanent hearing loss, those infants and toddlers with hearing loss secondary to OM may, in some states, be eligible under other portions of the regulation. If speech and language milestones are not met, these children may become eligible for IDEA Part C services through the provision of developmental language skills services. Children eligible for IDEA Part C may be afforded itinerant services by a teacher of the deaf and hard of hearing to reinforce basic, preacademic skills as well. It is noteworthy that such educators play an integral role in early intervention services for various types and degrees of hearing loss. A common misperception exists that individuals certified as teachers of the deaf and hard of hearing are relegated to teaching sign language or lip-reading when in fact they address all aspects of the insidious impact of hearing loss on educational access.

When children are ineligible for IDEA Part C early intervention services, the guidelines speak to several referrals to be made in the form of additional follow-up. This follow-up may include periodic monitoring of hearing status (every 3 months for those less than 1.5 years old and every 3–6 months for those up to 36 months of age), and careful monitoring of speech and language developmental milestones.

School Age

At the point of a child's third birthday, a new collaborative effort in service provision arises. The relationship between the child's school and the medical office takes shape. Twenty-first century families have a wide range of educational options for their children, including public schools, charter schools, private and parochial schools, and homeschooling. Although there remain some differences in how services in each of these arenas is provided, there are perhaps more similarities than differences. For the purpose of this article, the focus is on those schools that are bound by state and federal education laws in the public sector. It is at this juncture that there exists a significant difference in the delivery of services from the medical office to the classroom. This difference should not be viewed as a rift between the two but as an opportunity to collaborate with a clear understanding of how to make the necessary referrals for the continuum of services. **Table 3** shows the medical versus educational model of service provision.

Again, collaboration is the key to service provision for children in this age range, and both families and the medical community must develop an awareness of the services that are available in order that the children may have full access to services provided in the educational setting. Likewise, the educational community needs to be keenly aware of the services that are provided in the medical community. The process and the developing relationship must be bidirectional between the medical and health care service providers (physician and/or primary medical service provider and clinical audiologist) and the school-based professionals (educational audiologist, speech-language pathologist, classroom teacher, paraprofessionals, and so forth). Recommendations for educational modifications and accommodations should be made in

Table 3
Medical versus educational model of service provision
Collaboration is the key that unlocks services to children who may have medical needs that may also manifest in the educational realm. However, it may seem that physicians and the school-based professionals are speaking 2 different languages, both with the best interest of the patient/client at heart. The following is an analysis of the major differences between these 2 models. Gaining an understanding of how each part of the process varies enables professionals to request the appropriate service from the appropriate specialist using the appropriate procedural language. The result is more efficient and effective service provision.

Component of Service Provision	Medical Model	Educational Model (for Special Education and Related Services)
Identification of difficulty	Medical diagnosis based on standards of medical diagnoses known as ICD-10 set forth by the World Health Organization (https://www.cdc.gov/nchs/icd/icd10cm.htm)	1 of 13 Classifications based on IDEA 34 C.F.R. § 300 (2004) (http://idea.ed.gov/)
Testing terminology and time lines	Testing of disease or disorder and the process thereof is managed by the PCP or managing medical provider. Reevaluation/revision of diagnosis is only done if and when symptoms change	Testing for a suspected disabling condition is accomplished at the time of the initial referral for special education and related services and then revisited once every 3 y at a reevaluation planning meeting (https://www2.ed.gov/policy/speced/guid/idea/modelform-safeguards.pdf)
Testing may include (but is not limited to)	A battery of examinations and evaluations to arrive at the medical diagnosis. What testing and how many tests are done is a decision made solely at the discretion of the PCP, managing medical provider, or specialist	Social assessment, psychoeducational assessment, learning evaluation, speech and language evaluation, audiological evaluation, occupation and/or physical therapy evaluation, behavioral evaluation, pediatric neurologic evaluation, teacher evaluations. Which evaluations are chosen are based on a procedural meeting held by the school-based child study team
Outside assessments	Completed at the discretion of the PCP or managing medical provider based on the suspected diagnosis	May be introduced to the child study team, but the team is not obligated to accept an assessment or its recommendations. This assessment includes information provided to the school by the child's managing medical provider
Services provided through	A treatment plan managed by the PCP, managing medical provider, or medical specialist	The development of an IEP by a team of educational specialists, classroom staff, and the parent

(*continued on next page*)

Table 3 (*continued*)		
Component of Service Provision	**Medical Model**	**Educational Model (for Special Education and Related Services)**
Guidance for service provision provided by	American Medical Association, specialty medical practice associations, physician references, and standards/ guidelines of practice	US Department of Education and individual state education law
Eligibility for school-based services	A medical diagnosis does not automatically make a child eligible for service provision in the educational setting	A child is found eligible for special education and related services based on the results of the evaluations completed by the school-based child study team using the terminology inclusive of 1 of the 13 classifying conditions (http://idea.ed.gov/)
For school-based services to be provided	Contact needs to be made with a school-based SST who is then charged to prove a physical or mental impairment that substantially limits 1 or more major life activities (https://www.ada.gov/)	IEP team must determine manifestation of the disability in the educational setting (http://idea.ed.gov/)
Focus of related services	Among other related services, occupational, physical, and speech therapies may have a broader focus on the individual's whole environment	Some services, such as occupational and physical therapies, may be limited to skills that are educationally relevant and relate to a child's learning activities only
Fees	Cost of procedures either paid for through health insurance provider or out of pocket by the family based on CPT codes. (http://cptcodelist.com/)	No cost incurred by the family, based on the educational premise of free and appropriate public education (Pub.L. 93-112, 87 Stat. 355, enacted September 26, 1973)

Abbreviations: CPT, current procedural terminology; ICD; International Classification of Diseases; IEP, individual education program; PCP, primary care physician; SST, student support team.
  Reproduced with permission from Carol A. Ukstins and Deborah R. Welling.

collaboration with the educational audiologist, speech and language pathologist, and teachers in the school-based setting (**Table 4**).

Psychosocial Impact

As a sensory deficit, hearing loss can have far-reaching consequences; this is true regardless of cause, type, and degree of impairment. Notwithstanding, the potential negative impact of hearing loss on the quality of life and psychosocial aspects of functioning must also be addressed, particularly if the hearing loss has gone undiagnosed. Where children are concerned, it seems that parents may be more accurate in judging and reporting quality-of-life issues regarding functional health status rather than the less-observable emotional and social aspects of behavior.[24,25] Pain, fever, lack of sleep, changes in eating behaviors, attentional issues, and the like are symptoms

Table 4
Hearing loss (those degrees associated with otitis media with effusion) in education: a guide to service provision

| | Parent/Guardian Must Share Audiological Information with the School | | | |
| | Degree of Hearing Loss | | | |
	Fluctuating and Minimal Hearing Loss (<25 dB HL)	Mild Hearing Loss (25–40 dB HL)	Moderate Hearing Loss (40–55 dB HL)	Moderately Severe Hearing Loss (55–70 dB HL) Maximum Conductive Loss
Amplification HAT	CADS; Soundfield Technology	CADS; Soundfield Technology; totable device for small groups; personal HAT (if drainage does not accompany OME); personal amplification should be considered if condition is chronic	Personal HAT (if no drainage accompanies OME); totable device; personal amplification must be considered if condition is chronic, and integrated FM should be considered	Personal HAT (if no drainage accompanies OME); totable device; personal amplification must be considered if condition is chronic, and integrated FM should be strongly considered
Service eligibility (note: 504 eligibility criterion: a physical or mental disability which limits 1 or more major life activities; special education eligibility criteria: identification of 1 of the 13 classifying conditions that adversely effects educational performance)	SST for consideration of 504 plan; RTI in general education classroom; child may not be eligible for special education services solely on degree of hearing loss without demonstrating academic difficulties; may be ESLS if there are deficits resulting from auditory deprivation	SST for consideration of 504 plan; referral to CST if OME is chronic. May be eligible for special education and related services under classifying condition of auditorily impaired– hearing impaired: a hearing loss whether permanent or fluctuating that adversely effects educational performance	Evidence of academic difficulty may be more prevalent. If so, SST should be advised of hearing loss in order that accommodations and modifications are documented with the school. Parent may request (in writing) a direct referral to the CST for evaluation	Academic struggles are likely to be evident. All school personnel who come into contact with the child should be made aware of the hearing impairment for the safety and well-being of the child while in the physical building. Referral to the CST for evaluation is strongly recommended

(continued on next page)

Table 4
(continued)

	Parent/Guardian Must Share Audiological Information with the School Degree of Hearing Loss			
	Fluctuating and Minimal Hearing Loss (<25 dB HL)	Mild Hearing Loss (25–40 dB HL)	Moderate Hearing Loss (40–55 dB HL)	Moderately Severe Hearing Loss (55–70 dB HL) Maximum Conductive Loss
Listening challenges in the classroom	Difficulty following soft speech; difficulty following classroom conversations with rapid exchange of information; difficulty distinguishing subtle cues in a conversation (sarcasm, jokes, multiple meanings; and so forth); seems to lose focus or fatigue easily	Without amplification, may miss up to 40% of instruction in a classroom; easily distracted by background noise; listening fatigue is evident; daydreaming or phasing out during classroom instruction may be reported; child is described as being off-topic during classroom discussions; reading/writing and spelling are affected	Without amplification, 50%–75% of information may be missed or heard inaccurately; significant receptive and expressive language deficits may manifest in delayed reading and writing skills; inattention can be mistaken for behavioral attention issues; child may begin to act out in class; children may socially isolate themselves or be described as socially awkward	Without the use of amplification; close to 100% of average conversational speech may not be heard; significant expressive and receptive language deficits, articulation errors, as well as significant academic delays are likely to be identified; child may have poor socialization skills caused by the inability to effectively communicate with peers
School staff who may be involved in service provision	School nurse; teacher; classroom paraprofessional staff; SST; possible observation by an SLP; review of results by an educational audiologist	School nurse; teacher; classroom paraprofessional staff; SST; CST including the SLP and educational audiologist	SST; general education teacher; push-in RTI services; CST including SLP and educational audiologist; itinerate services of a TODHH	General education teacher; TODHH; CST including SLP and educational audiologist

Classroom accommodations (recommendations for learning the same material in the classroom and meeting the same expectations as their classmates)	Visual supplements to auditory information; strategic seating; buddy system for note-taking; step-by-step directions; built in downtime after auditory tasks; extended test-taking time	All of previous and obtain child's visual attention before speaking with a tap or by calling the child by name; extended time to complete assignments; routine checks for understanding of concepts	All of previous and classroom noise/reverberation reduction; captioning of multimedia; allow extra time for processing of auditory information; repeating and/or rephrasing information; frequent checks for academic understanding	All of previous and itinerate TODHH services to promote communication access; assign note taker; implement speech-to-text software; alternative placement options may need to be explored if child is struggling academically
Classroom modifications (change to what the student is taught or expected to learn)	Provide supplemental materials; preteach new vocabulary; pretutoring and/or posttutoring of academic information	All of previous and reading assistance for test-taking; separate setting for test-taking; reduce demands for homework assignments (shorter length; fewer practice items)	All of previous and reduce quantity of test materials; consider alternative testing methods; modification of written assignments; tutoring or additional instruction by a TODHH	All of previous and implement alternative teaching methods to accommodate reduced auditory access; direct instruction by a TODHH; increased student/teacher ratio or add additional support staff to assist with work completion

Each child's condition and needs are unique. Services within the school are based on strict state and federal guidelines and may vary from school district to school district. This information is provided to expose readers to service, that may be available to students experiencing educational difficulty secondary to OME and hearing loss.

Abbreviations: CADS, classroom audio distribution system; CST, child student team; ESLS, eligible for speech and language services; HAT, hearing assistance technology; SLP, speech-language pathologist; TODHH, teacher of the deaf and hard of hearing.

Reproduced with permission from Carol A. Ukstins and Deborah R. Welling.

more easily recognized and thus brought to the attention of medical service providers. However, the social-emotional aspects manifesting from the hearing loss may be more prevalent in social settings, such as the classroom and/or the playground. As a result, parents or guardians may be less likely to report these behaviors. Difficulty establishing peer relationships, the inability to produce work when assigned to small groups, reduced auditory attention, decreased or inappropriate social behaviors, and physical manifestation of frustration rather than using conventional words are behaviors and symptoms more likely to be reported by teachers or secondary caregivers. The secondary and tertiary effects of undetected and untreated hearing loss have the potential to be extensive, not only for individuals who are hard of hearing but for those persons' families and loved ones as well.

Karen Anderson, a prominent educational audiologist, has published extensively on this topic. Interested readers may wish to access http://successforkidswith hearingloss.com/relationship-hl-listen-learn/ for further information and resources.

SUMMARY

The treatment continuum of OME cannot stop with the medical provider. The impact OME has (in all of its stages) on hearing, listening, learning, and psychosocial health must be addressed when developing an appropriate treatment plan. The medical provider is in charge of the diagnosis and management of the disorder, but it is only with the collaborative and interprofessional efforts of a team-based approach, including the clinical audiologist, speech-language pathologist, educational audiologist, as well as those professionals within the educational setting, that the best patient outcomes for individuals with OME will be realized.

REFERENCES

1. Rosenfeld RM, Shin JJ, Schwartz SR, et al. Clinical practice guideline: otitis media with effusion (update). Otolaryngol Head Neck Surg 2016;154(1):1–41.
2. Bluestone CD, Gates GA, Klein JO, et al. Definitions, terminology, and classification of otitis media. Ann Otol Rhinol Laryngol 2002;Part 2 of 2(111):8–18.
3. Lieberthal AS, Carroll AE, Chonmaitree T. The diagnosis and management of acute otitis media pediatrics 2013;131:e964–9. Available at: https://www.ncbi.nlm.nih.gov/pubmed/2349909. Accessed April 11, 2017.
4. Fourgner V, Korvel-Hanquist A, Koch A, et al. Early childhood otitis media and later school performance – a prospective cohort study of associations. Int J Otorhinolaryngol 2017;94:87–94.
5. Avnstorp MB, Homoe P, Bjerregaard P, et al. Chronic suppurative otitis media, middle ear pathology and corresponding hearing loss in a cohort of Greenlandic children. Int J Pediatr Otorhinolaryngol 2016;83:148–53.
6. Yehudai N, Most T, Luntz M. Risk factors for sensorineural hearing loss in pediatric chronic otitis media. Int J Pediatr Otorhinolaryngol 2015;79:26–30.
7. Tiido M, Stiles D. Cochlear damage and otitis media. Audiol Today 2013;25(1):62–4.
8. DaCosta SS, Rosito LPS, Dornelles C. Sensorineural hearing loss in patients with chronic otitis media. Eur Arch Otorhinolaryngol 2009;266:221–4.
9. Winiger AM, Alexander JM, Diefendorf AO. Minimal hearing loss: from failure-based approach to evidence-based practice. Am J Audiol 2016;25(3):232–45.
10. Whitton JP, Polley DB. Ear infections today, "Lazy Ear" tomorrow? Audiol Today 2012;24(4):32–7.

11. Shetty HN, Koonoor V. Sensory deprivation due to otitis media episodes in early childhood and its effect at later age: a psychoacoustic and speech perception measure. Int J Pediatr Otorhinolaryngol 2016;90:181–7.
12. Sandeep M, Jayaram M. Effect of early otitis media on speech identification. Aust New Zeal J Audiol 2008;30(1):38–49.
13. Daud MK, Noor RM, Rahman NA, et al. The effect of mild hearing loss on academic performance in primary school children. Int J Pediatr Otorhinolaryngol 2010;74:67–70.
14. Cone BK, Wake M, Tobin S, et al. Slight-mild sensorineural hearing loss in children: audiometric, clinical, and risk factor profiles. Ear Hear 2010;31(2):202–12.
15. Knobel KAB, Lima MCMP. Are parents aware of their children's hearing complaints? Braz J Otorhinolaryngol 2012;78(5):27–37.
16. Lo PSY, Tong MCF, Wong EMC, et al. Parental suspicion of hearing loss in children with otitis media with effusion. Eur J Pediatr 2006;165:851–7.
17. Hall JW. Objective assessment of infant hearing: essential for early intervention. J Hear Sci 2016;6(2):9–25.
18. Schriberg LD, Freil-Patti S, Flipsen P Jr, et al. Otitis media, fluctuant hearing loss, and speech-language outcomes: a preliminary structural equation model. J Speech Lang Hear Res 2000;43:100–20.
19. Roberts JE, Rosenfeld RM, Zeisel SA. Otitis media and speech and language: a meta-analysis of prospective studies. Pediatrics 2004;113(3):238–48.
20. Winskel H. The effects of an early history of otitis media on children's language and literacy skill development. Br J Educ Psychol 2006;76:727–44.
21. Perigoe CB, Paterson MM. Understanding auditory development and the child with hearing loss. In: Welling DR, Ukstins CA, editors. Fundamentals of audiology for the speech-language pathologist. Burlington (MA): Jones & Bartlett; 2015.
22. Individuals with Disabilities Education Act. 2004. PL 108 – 446, 20 USC 1400 note. 118. Stat. 2648. Available at: http://www.ed.gov/policy.
23. Individuals with Disabilities Education Act. 2004. PL 108 – 446, 20 USC 1432. Note. 118. Stat. 2744. Available at: http://www.law.cornell.edu/uscode/text/20/1432.
24. Brouwer CNM, Maille AR, Rovers MM, et al. Health-related quality of life in children with otitis media. Int J Pediatr Otorhinolaryngol 2005;69:1031–41.
25. Upton P, Lawford J, Eiser C. Parent-child agreement across child health-related quality of life instruments: a review of the literature. Qual Life Res 2008;17:895–913.

Using the International Classification of Functioning, Disability and Health Framework to Achieve Interprofessional Functional Outcomes for Young Children

A Speech-Language Pathology Perspective

Lemmietta G. McNeilly, PhD

KEYWORDS

- Functional outcomes • Young children
- International Classification of Functioning, Disability and Health framework
- Speech and language disorders • Activities and participation of children

KEY POINTS

- The International Classification of Functioning, Disability and Health (ICF) Framework is used to write functional goals.
- Functional goals are set for young children with communication disorders.
- Interprofessional collaboration can benefit from the ICF framework.

INTERNATIONAL CLASSIFICATION OF FUNCTIONING, DISABILITY, AND HEALTH

The World Health Organization (WHO) launched the International Classification of Functioning, Disability and Health (ICF), a comprehensive coding system that views functioning and disability as a conceptual framework and a common language between all professions, focusing primarily on adults.[1–4] In 2007, the WHO published a new internationally agreed-upon comprehensive classification system based on the ICD to assess the health of children and youth in the context of their developmental stages and living environments. The International Classification of Functioning, Disability and Health for Children and Youth (ICF-CY) verifies the importance of

Disclosure Statement: No competing interests to disclose.
Speech-Language Pathology, American Speech-Language-Hearing Association, 2200 Research Boulevard, #229, Rockville, MD 20850-3289, USA
E-mail address: Lmcneilly@asha.org

describing children's health using a methodology that applies codes for bodily functions and structures, activities and participation, and environmental factors that either limit or help children to function in an array of everyday activities. In 2012, the WHO merged the ICF and the ICF-CY to enhance usage for the transition across the life span. The ICF is the WHO framework that measures health and disability at both individual and population levels. The WHO Disability Assessment Schedule (WHODAS 2.0) was developed as a collaborative international approach aimed at assessing health status and disability across various cultures and settings.

FUNCTIONAL GOAL WRITING USING THE INTERNATIONAL CLASSIFICATION OF FUNCTIONING, DISABILITY AND HEALTH FRAMEWORK

Functional goals are written for individuals and target their ability to participate in daily living environments across settings including home, school, and community. The focus is not on the impairment or disorder but on the participation in activities of daily living.

Speech-language pathologists (SLPs) need to obtain knowledge and skills and become competent to teach information to others including graduate clinicians, children, and families regarding the ICF framework for writing functional goals for children. Additionally, SLPs need to be competent in the delivery of services after assessing a child's communication skills and limitations and successes interacting with others within their daily living environments. Graduate programs can infuse the ICF framework within clinical practicum coursework. Graduate students need to acquire the ability to use the ICF framework as an assessment component to evaluate a child's speech, language and social skills, and limitations exhibited during communication interactions and to develop appropriate functional goals for children's needs.

The American Speech-Language-Hearing Association's (ASHA) Scope of Practice in Speech-Language Pathology describes the diagnostic categories that are consistent with relevant diagnostic categories in the ICF framework.[5–9] The ICF framework is useful in describing the SLP's role in prevention, assessment, and habilitation/rehabilitation of communication and swallowing disorders. The framework consists of 2 components: health conditions and contextual factors.

HEALTH CONDITIONS
Body Functions and Structures

These involve the anatomy and physiology of the human body. Relevant examples in speech-language pathology include craniofacial anomaly, vocal fold paralysis, cerebral palsy, stuttering, and language impairment.

Activity and Participation

Activity refers to the execution of a task or action. Participation is the involvement in a life situation. Relevant examples in speech-language pathology include difficulties with swallowing safely for independent feeding, participating actively in class, understanding a medical prescription, and accessing the general education curriculum.

CONTEXTUAL FACTORS
Environmental Factors

These comprise the physical, social, and attitudinal environments in which people live and conduct their lives. Relevant examples in speech-language pathology include the role of the communication partner in augmentative and alternative communication (AAC), the influence of classroom acoustics on communication, and the impact of institutional dining environments on individuals' ability to safely maintain nutrition and hydration.

Personal Factors

These refer to the internal influences on an individual's functioning and disability and are not part of the health condition. Personal factors may include, but are not limited to, age, gender, ethnicity, educational level, social background, and profession. Relevant examples in speech-language pathology might include an individual's background or culture, if one or both influence his or her reaction to communication or swallowing.

The framework in speech-language pathology encompasses these health conditions and contextual factors across individuals and populations. **Fig. 1** illustrates the interaction of the various components of the ICF framework. The health condition component is expressed on a continuum of functioning. On 1 end of the continuum is intact functioning; at the opposite end of the continuum is completely compromised function. The contextual factors interact with each other and with the health conditions and may serve as facilitators or barriers to functioning. SLPs influence contextual factors through education and advocacy efforts at local, state, and national levels.

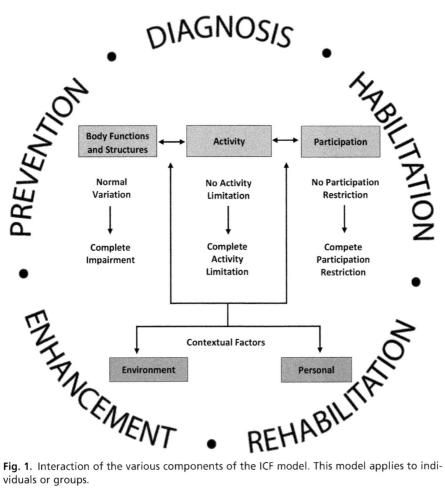

Fig. 1. Interaction of the various components of the ICF model. This model applies to individuals or groups.

The ICF-CY is based on the original ICF framework, and provides a biopsychosocial framework that uses universal language to address health concerns that are specifically relevant to infants, toddlers, children, and adolescents. The ICF-CY framework is comprised of 2 parts: (1) functioning and disability and (2) contextual factors that influence children's health.[10] The functioning and disability section consists of 2 components: body functions and structures, and activities and participation. Contextual factors include environmental and personal factors.[10] Within the ICF-CY framework, a child's functioning and disability are viewed as being in dynamic interaction between health conditions and contextual factors.

There are significant debates in the literature about whether to distinguish between the activities and participation components of the ICF framework.[11,12] For this reason, the WHO identified 4 options that can be used to interpret the relationship between activities and participation.[3]

COMMUNICATION DISORDERS

Communication disorders include specific disorders in speech, language, feeding, and swallowing. Children with these disorders often exhibit limitations in their abilities to communicate with diverse individuals in different environments. Intervention is designed to improve functional outcomes that will result in greater successful participation communicating with peers and adults at home, school, and in the community.

ASSESSMENT

The assessment of children while they participate in daily functioning depends on the framework used to conceptualize functioning and disability. The Pediatric Evaluation of Disability Inventory (PEDI), the study conducted by Ostensjo, Bjorbakmo, Carlberg, and Vollestad, used the ICF framework as a framework of functioning and disability that could be used to compare the measurement constructs and the content of different outcome measurements. This methodology examined the conceptual basis and the content of the PEDI using the ICF framework. The study systematically collected and analyzed phrases that described the conceptual basis of the PEDI scales and of the ICF classifications for comparison. The analyses indicated that the conceptual basis of the PEDI scales matched the ICF concepts of activity, participation, and environmental factors. Both the PEDI and the ICF framework used the constructs of capacity and performance, but differed in how these constructs were operationalized. The classification of the functional skills scales showed that the PEDI was a measure of activities and participation. The analyses indicated that the ICF can serve as a conceptual framework to clarify the measurement construct of the PEDI scales, and as taxonomy to describe and clarify the item content of the functional skills scales. Both as a framework and taxonomy, the ICF showed limitations in addressing a young child's functioning.[13]

COMMUNICATION PERFORMANCE

The assessment of a child's communication performance with multiple communication partners can be assessed in multiple environments including at home, school, and in the community. Effective communication is important and of significant value to families. Several studies have reviewed communication skills of different populations of children, including children with Down syndrome, traumatic brain injury (TBI), and a review study of several types of communication disorders including autism spectrum disorder and language disorders. A synopsis of these studies reveals the value of the ICF framework in assessment and development of functional treatment goals.

An ICF-CY based multiple-case study of the communication performance of young children with Down syndrome was reported in the Netherlands. Enhancing communication performance skills may help children with Down syndrome to expand their participation in different daily living situations. It is a clinical challenge for speech-language pathologists to disentangle various mechanisms that contribute to the language and communication problems encountered by children. In this study, the ICF-CY framework was used to classify factors that contributed to communication performance in a multiple-case study of 6 young children with Down syndrome. Within a comprehensive assessment, individual and environmental facilitators and barriers were identified that led to an integrative profile of communication performance (IPCP) for each child. These 6 children shared a developmental, and/or expressive vocabulary age and/or level of communicative intent; the children faced similar but unique personal and environmental factors that impacted their communication performance. The data revealed that a combination of different factors may have led to the same language outcomes and vice versa, based on a unique pattern of interdependency of ICF-CY domains. Planning speech-language pathologist interventions that enhance communication performance in children with Down syndrome should be based on a comprehensive view of the competencies and limitations presented by an individual child and the communication partners. The evaluation should address facilitators and barriers in body functions, structures, activities, participation, and environment, with a specific focus on individual strengths. The ICF-CY is a useful framework for constructing an IPCP that serves this purpose.[14]

MEASURING HEALTH OUTCOMES

Health services are increasing their focus on measuring outcomes. Various elements contribute to the value of outcome measures. The outcomes should be valued by patients and caregivers, be consistent with targets by health professionals, and have robust measurement properties. The aim of the study by Morris and colleagues[15] was twofold (1) to seek a shared vision between families and clinicians regarding key aspects of health as outcomes, and (2) to appraise which multidimensional patient-reported outcome measures (PROMs) could be used to assess salient health domains.

The study method included relevant outcomes identified from

1. Qualitative research with children and young people with neurologic disability and parent caregivers
2. Delphi survey with health professionals
3. Systematic review of PROMs

The International Classification of Functioning Disability and Health provided a common language to code aspects of health. A subset of stakeholders participated in a prioritization meeting incorporating a Q-sorting task to discuss and rank aspects of health. Thirty-three pertinent aspects of health were identified. Fifteen stakeholders from the qualitative and Delphi studies participated in the prioritization meeting: 3 young people, 5 parent caregivers, and 7 health professionals. The aspects of health that were more important for families and targets for health professionals included: communication, emotional wellbeing, pain, sleep, mobility, self-care, independence, mental health, community and social life, behavior, toileting, and safety. The available PROMs measured many aspects of health in the ICF; no single PROM captured all the key domains prioritized for children and young people with neurologic disability. The paucity of scales that assess communication was notable. Conclusions of this study proposed a core suite of key outcome domains for children with neurologic disability that could be used in evaluative research and as health service performance indicators. Future work could appraise domain-specific PROMs for these aspects of health; a single measure assessing the key aspects of health that could be applied across pediatric neurologic disability still needs to be developed.[15]

TRAUMATIC BRAIN INJURY INTERVENTION

The role of contextual factors in the rehabilitation of adolescent survivors of TBI was investigated in the study by Ciccia and Threats.[16] Research in TBI intervention has identified the benefits of contextualized, embedded, functionally based approaches to maximize treatment outcomes. An essential component of contextualized intervention was the direct and purposeful consideration of the broader context, in which the person with TBI functioned. Systematic consideration of contextual factors remains limited in research and clinical practice. The purposes of this modified narrative review were

To provide a succinct review of the available literature regarding the contextual factors specific to adolescent survivors of TBI

To connect these contextual factors to the direct long-term management of TBI and to identify their potential impact on outcome

To highlight areas that were open to research and clinical advances that could enhance positive outcomes for adolescent survivors of TBI[16]

The framework of the ICF-CY[10] served as the foundation for this review. A systematic literature search was conducted using databases and hand searches. Twenty-five original research articles, 8 review papers, and 4 expert opinion papers met inclusion and exclusion criteria and were included in the final review. The body of research specifically focused on contextual factors is an emerging area. Early findings indicated that a focus on the direct modification of contextual factors was promising for the facilitation of positive outcomes into the chronic phase of management for adolescents who have survived a TBI. The contextual factors included in this review were the overall ability of the school to support a student after the TBI, family psychosocial risk (sibling/sibling relationships/stress/burden/support), coping styles of the TBI survivor and his or her caregivers, and socioeconomic status of the family. Given the promise of these findings, research and clinical application efforts should be focused on identifying well-prescribed rehabilitation paradigms that modify contextual factors throughout the recovery process. The results of this modified narrative review provided an initial summary of the available evidence that addressed contextual factors in the rehabilitation process for adolescents with TBI. This is an area that exhibits potential to improve long-term outcome for survivors of adolescent TBI.[16]

A review article identified current methods for evaluating speech-language outcomes of preschoolers with communication disorders.[17] The review identified current practices for evaluating speech-language outcomes for preschoolers with communication disorders. Most outcomes in the review were evaluated for the ICF-CY body functions and activities components, with fewer evaluating outcomes related to the participation component. Typically, speech-language pathologists address participation-based issues in therapy. The authors encouraged practicing clinicians to use some of the broadly focused, valid, and reliable participation-based outcome measures that were identified in the review.

Including a participation-based outcome assessment tool in addition to those focused on the body functions and activities components can provide clinicians with a bigger picture of how interventions affect children and families in their everyday lives. Traditionally, speech-language pathologists engage in correction of speech and language errors within the treatment sessions; parents are more interested in how their child's communication disorder affects his or her ability to participate in school and with peers.[18] Measuring participation-based outcomes may be more meaningful to families and may facilitate conversations related to goal setting and therapy using family-friendly language.

The inclusion of participation-based outcomes would also assist health care organizations with evaluating the impacts of speech-language interventions for children with all types of communication disorders. This would be valuable, as it is generally difficult to compare outcomes for children with different types of disorders (eg, comparing outcomes for children with speech sound disorders vs receptive language delays). Participation-based outcomes would be more meaningful for individuals with a range of communication impairments also.[19] Organizations would be able to show meaningful changes for large groups of children, and present information in family friendly language rather than using professional jargon.

The American Speech-Language-Hearing Association (ASHA) Scope of Practice in Speech-Language Pathology[5] emphasizes the need for continued commitment to the evaluation of outcomes for all components of the ICF, including participation. Although the ICF has been in use since 2001 and has been included in versions of the Scope of Practice in Speech-Language Pathology since 2007, there is a paucity of participation-based outcomes research in the field. The authors of this article encourage others to include meaningful participation-based outcomes in future research studies. Additionally, future research and practice to include these measures for the purpose of facilitating measurement of meaningful life changes that result from children's participation in speech-language interventions beyond the changes associated with the body functions and activities is necessary.

INTERPROFESSIONAL SERVICE DELIVERY

Speech-language pathologists work collaboratively with other health professionals and family members to assess and execute functional goals that will successfully target the successful participation for children in the home, school and community environments. Interprofessional practice (IPP) is enhanced using the ICF framework. It allows the use of a classification system that covers all aspects of an individual, and professionals would share the tool for assessment and goal writing. It is important for parents and family members to express their targets and understand how they can facilitate the child's progress and ultimate achievement of the targeted outcomes for communication.

Young children enrolled in early intervention programs are often seen outside of the home and need to learn to communicate effectively with peers and other adults in new settings. Having goals that only focus on the specific types of sounds that they have difficulty producing or learning new words outside of the understanding of the communication needs within both the home and the early intervention center may not yield the desired results. Using the ICF framework to write functional goals that are appropriate for the settings and communication situations will help each of the team members to actively reinforce the desired functional goals in naturalistic ways.

Clinicians working in schools can also benefit from using the ICF framework to develop goals with educational relevance and enhance the student's successful communication with peers and teachers in the classroom, cafeteria, and traveling to and from school. Students are required to communicate about a variety of topics and with different communication partners. Social communication skills are critical in developing friendships and relationships with others. The ICF framework is a tool that facilitates interprofessional collaboration with other professionals to address the student's needs.

Community-based services are additional opportunities for children and families to communicate in a variety of ways with multiple partners. The limitations exhibited can be targeted to maximize successful participation in communication interactions with others. Speech-language pathologists can see firsthand the issues and develop strategies that are practical and achieve the desired functional outcomes for the child and family.

American Speech-Language-Hearing Association Resources

There are resources regarding how to use the ICF framework on the ASHA Web site. Such resources include 4 webinars, an overview of the ICF framework, and interprofessional collaborative practice and person-centered care using the ICF framework with ICF case studies in speech-language pathology, occupational therapy and physical therapy. Templates of functional goal writing using the ICF for at least 12 different communication disorders are also available at http://www.asha.org/slp/icf/.

The ASHA site includes 2 functional goal writing samples using the ICF framework

- Specific language impairment - http://www.asha.org/uploadedFiles/ICF-Specific-Language-Impairment.pdf
- Speech sound disorder - http://www.asha.org/uploadedFiles/ICF-Speech-Sound-Disorder.pdf

SUMMARY

Ultimately, outcomes should be the goal of all intervention efforts, and the ICF framework helps to facilitate successful functional outcomes for children across daily living environments. The ICF framework is an ideal tool that many health care professionals can utilize to write functional goals and assess the child's participation in multiple communication interactions. One critical element of the ICF-CY sometimes overlooked is evaluating the effectiveness of clinical intervention. Health care providers who take the time to learn how to use the ICF will find that the value gained in functional patient outcomes will be well worth the investment.

Pediatricians serve as leaders of health care teams and have a significant role in selecting appropriate tools for assessing children and monitoring their functional performance. There are opportunities for more clinical teams within the United States to consider the utility of the ICF as a framework for assessing and monitoring the functional outcomes of children.

A study of children receiving Florida Medicaid benefits conducted to develop item banks that linked pediatric quality-of-life instruments utilized the ICF-CY framework.[20] The framework facilitated comparison of item concepts from 3 instruments to determine the most salient items for assessing a pediatric population. The results concluded that the ICF-CY is a useful framework for comparing the concepts of items from 3 pediatric legacy instruments. It suggested its utility for both researchers and clinical practice.

There are additional studies of pediatricians utilizing the ICF-CY framework in clinical rehabilitation in Europe. A study completed in Italy[21] investigated the effect of implementation of the ICF-CY on team members and families for framing rehabilitation in a pediatric outpatient clinic for adolescents with cerebral palsy and complex medical conditions. The results indicated that the framework provided a language and bio-psycho-social model about which each of the stakeholders had favorable feedback regarding the ICF-CY. Pediatricians, speech-language pathologists, physical therapists, and other members of health care service delivery teams should consider the merits of the ICF-CF framework.

REFERENCES

1. Threats TT. WHO's international classification of functioning, disability, and health: a framework for clinical and research outcomes. In: Golper LAC, Frattali CM, editors. Outcomes in speech-language pathology. 2nd edition. New York: Thieme; 2013. p. 58–72.

2. World Health Organization. International classification of functioning, disability and health. Geneva (Switzerland): Author; 2014. Available at: www.who.int/classifications/icf/en/gol.

3. World Health Organization. International classification of functioning, disability and health. Geneva (Switzerland): Author; 2001.

4. World Health Organization. Merger of the ICF and ICF-CY. 2012. Available at: http://www.who.int/classifications/icf/whoficresolution2012icfcy.pdf?ua=1. Accessed October 28, 2017.

5. American Speech-Language-Hearing Association. Scope of practice in speech-language pathology [Scope of practice]. 2016. Available at: http://www.asha.org/policy. Accessed October 28, 2017.

6. Skarakis-Doyle E, Doyle P. The ICF as a framework for interdisciplinary doctoral education in rehabilitation: implications for speech-language pathology. Int J Speech Lang Pathol 2008;10:83–91.

7. McLeod S, Threats T. The ICF-CY and children with communication disabilities. Int J Speech Lang Pathol 2008;10:92–109.

8. McCormack J, McLeod S, Harrison L, et al. The impact of speech impairment in early childhood: investigating parents' and speech-language pathologists' perspectives using the ICF-CY. J Commun Disord 2010;43:378–96.

9. McLeod S, McCormack J. Application of the ICF and the ICF–Children and Youth in children with speech impairment. Semin Speech Lang 2007;28:254–64.

10. World Health Organization. International classification of functioning, disability and health–children and youth version. Geneva (Switzerland): Author; 2007.

11. Threats T, Worrall L. Classifying communication disability using the ICF. Advances in Speech-Language Pathology 2004;6:53–62.

12. Washington KN. Using the ICF within speech-language pathology: application to developmental language impairment. Advances in Speech-Language Pathology 2007;9:242–55, doc.

13. Ostensjo S, Bjorbakmo W, Carlberg E, et al. Assessment of everyday functioning in young children with disabilities: an ICF-based analysis of concepts and content of the Pediatric Evaluation of Disability Inventory (PEDI). Disabil Rehabil 2006;28(8):489–504.

14. Deckers SM, Van Zaalen Y, Stoep J, et al. Communication performance of children with Down Syndrome: an ICF-CY based multiple case study. Child Lang Teach Ther 2016;32(3):293–311.

15. Morris C, Janssens A, Shilling V, et al. Meaningful health outcomes for paediatric neurodisability: stakeholder prioritisation and appropriateness of patient reported outcome measures. Health Qual Life Outcomes 2015;13(1):87.
16. Ciccia AH, Threats T. Role of contextual factors in the rehabilitation of adolescent survivors of traumatic brain injury: emerging concepts identified through modified narrative review. Int J Lang Commun Disord 2015;50(4):436–51.
17. Cunningham BJ, Washington K, Binns A, et al. Current methods of evaluating speech-language outcomes for preschoolers with communication disorders: a scoping review using the ICF-CY. J Speech Lang Hear Res 2017;60:447–64.
18. Thomas-Stonell N, Oddson B, Robertson B, et al. Predicted and observed outcomes in preschool children following speech and language treatment: 11. Parent and clinician perspectives. J Commun Disord 2009;42:29–42.
19. Cieza A, Anczewska M, Ayuso-Mateos JL, et al, PARADISE Consortium. Understanding the impact of brain disorders: towards a "horizontal epidemiology" of psychosocial difficulties and their determinants. PLoS One 2015;10(9):e0136271.
20. Gandhi P, Thompson LS, Tuli SY, et al. Developing item banks for measuring pediatric generic health-related quality of life: an application of the international classification of functioning, disability and health for children and youth and item response theory. PLoS One 2014;9(9):e107771.
21. Martinuzzi A, De Polo G, Bortolot S, et al. Pediatric neurorehabilitation and the ICF. NeuroRehabilitation 2015;36:31–6.

Developmental and Interprofessional Care of the Preterm Infant

Neonatal Intensive Care Unit Through High-Risk Infant Follow-up

Hildy S. Lipner, MA, CCC/SLP[a],*, Randye F. Huron, MS, MD[b]

KEYWORDS

- Preterm infants • Developmental care • Neonatal intensive care unit environment
- Oral feeding • Neurodevelopment • Developmental monitoring • Early intervention

KEY POINTS

- Opportunities to improve cognitive, neuropsychological, and behavioral outcomes for preterm infants begin in the neonatal intensive care unit (NICU).
- Developmental care in the NICU includes changes in the delivery of medical and physical care, supportive handling techniques, infant-led oral feeding practices, and adaptations to the environment that limit infant stress and enhance self-regulation.
- The population of very low birth weight preterm infants is at highest risk for difficulties with transition to oral feeding and for persisting oral feeding challenges that continue to require skilled therapeutic assistance after discharge.
- Proactive developmental monitoring and implementation of timely therapeutic and educational early intervention services are essential to continue to support optimal outcomes for preterm infants.

DEVELOPMENTAL CARE OF THE PRETERM INFANT: NEONATAL INTENSIVE CARE UNIT THROUGH HIGH-RISK INFANT FOLLOW-UP

According to the National Vital Statistics Report published by the US Centers for Disease Control and Prevention (CDC) in January 2017,[1] the preterm birth rate in the United States in 2015, covering all infants born less than 37 weeks, was 9.63%, a

The authors have no commercial or financial conflicts to disclose and have received no financial compensation for producing this material.

[a] Pediatric Speech Pathology, Institute for Child Development, Joseph M. Sanzari Children's Hospital, Hackensack University Medical Center, 30 Prospect Avenue, Hackensack, NJ 07601, USA; [b] Developmental and Behavioral Pediatrics, Institute for Child Development, Joseph M. Sanzari Children's Hospital, Hackensack University Medical Center, 30 Prospect Avenue, Hackensack, NJ 07601, USA

* Corresponding author.

E-mail address: hildy.lipner@hackensackmeridian.org

Pediatr Clin N Am 65 (2018) 135–141
https://doi.org/10.1016/j.pcl.2017.08.026
0031-3955/18/© 2017 Elsevier Inc. All rights reserved.
pediatric.theclinics.com

slight increase from 9.57% in 2014. The percentage of infants classified as low birth-weight (<2500 g) also rose slightly, from 8.00% to 8.07%, from 2014 to 2015. Infants classified as moderately low birthweight (1500–2499 g) increased from 6.60% to 6.67%, while the very low birthweight rate (<1500 g) remained stable at 1.40%. Advances in medical intervention and treatment have improved the survival of premature infants including the population of very low birth-weight infants, placing an ever-growing emphasis on improving the long-term developmental outcomes for this most vulnerable pediatric population.

In 1986, Public Law 99-457 was enacted to provide access to federal funding, so that each individual state could begin implementation of early intervention programs for at-risk children from birth to 5 years of age. At the same time, research by Als was initiated to determine if changes made even earlier during infant care in the neonatal intensive care unit (NICU) could have a long-lasting positive impact on the cognitive and behavioral outcomes of premature infants.[2,3]

Als studied the impact of the environment in the NICU on the developing brain of the premature infant and proposed a framework for interpreting and responding to an infant's behavioral cues and providing care-based interventions to address the noxious effects of environmental stress upon the neonate.[4–6] Multiple studies have demonstrated the positive effects of these "developmental interventions" in the NICU upon brain structure, motor organization and development, and longer-term cognitive and behavior outcomes.[7–13]

This article proposes that establishing a continuum of services beginning in the NICU and transitioning through careful developmental and interprofessional follow-up and availability of early therapeutic and educational interventions following discharge would best support the achievement of optimal outcomes for premature infants. Current protocols followed at the Joseph M. Sanzari Children's Hospital at Hackensack University Medical Center have been utilized for illustrative purposes.

Getting off to a Good Start: Implementing Developmental Care in the Neonatal Intensive Care Unit

In the authors' NICU, developmental care relates to

- Practices and protocols guiding medical interventions
- Approaches to physical care
- Guidelines for positioning and handling
- Noise and lighting control
- Relationship building and parental participation in infant care
- Oral feeding practices

The interprofessional team includes neonatologists, physician assistants, advanced practice and bedside neonatal nurses, physical and occupational therapists, speech-language pathologists, child life specialists, and social workers.

Emphasis on comfort care during medical procedures to minimize pain and stress includes providing non-nutritive sucking to promote calming and neurologic organization paired with sucrose, as well as hand hugging (cradling of the head with the hands). Nursing staff, child life specialists, and parents when appropriate can be present to provide comfort care during medical procedures. Clustering physical care promotes periods of uninterrupted rest/sleep and energy conservation. Physical and occupational therapists provide guidance for nursing and parents with respect to provision of an individualized developmental care plan to reduce environmental stress. Optimal positioning for postural support, skull shaping and energy conservation, as well as, handling techniques that encourage positive positional transitions are taught. Parents are taught to identify their infant's behavior cues to establish early parental confidence and success in meeting infant's needs and to enhance the infant's self-regulatory capabilities.

In the authors' NICU, every effort is made to introduce direct skin-to-skin contact with parents as soon as the infant is deemed medically stable to accommodate transfer from the isolette. Kangaroo Care, where the infant is laid directly against the parent's unclothed chest, has been found to improve temperature regulation, oxygen saturation, and sleep, as well as, positively initiate the parent-infant bonding process.[14–16] Both mothers and fathers are encouraged to participate in Kangaroo Care. Nursing staff members provide parents with education regarding the positive effects of Kangaroo Care, encourage participation, and assuage parental fears. It can sometimes take the coordination of nurse, respiratory therapist, and an occupational or physical therapist to accomplish a successful transfer.

Steps are taken to minimize noise and provide positive auditory stimulation at appropriate decibel levels. Parents are encouraged to talk and read to their infants and can make voice recordings to be played when mother and father cannot be present. The authors' NICU has also experimented with periods of live classical music provided by a child life/music therapist to promote calming and stress reduction for infants, parents, and staff.[17] Harsh overhead bright lighting is avoided, unless medically necessary. Dimmers on all light switches provide the opportunity to situationally alter lighting. Older infants can be transitioned to corner room areas with windows, allowing the opportunity for exposure to natural light.[18]

Initiating oral feeding is a milestone event in the life of a premature infant and his or her parents. The authors' NICU has adopted an infant-led approach to oral feeding based upon the Infant Driven Feeding Protocol developed by Ludwig and Waitzman.[19] This approach emphasizes and measures the "quality" of oral feeding ability as opposed to quantity of intake, provides a unified vocabulary for both NICU staff and parents to use when discussing oral feeding and encourages parental competence, confidence, and independence while feeding their baby. Trained staff help to teach parents to identify well-defined infant behavioral cues to determine infant "readiness" to initiate oral feeding, as well as cues that indicate infant "stress" and the need to stop a feeding. Assessment by a speech-language pathologist is available to assist with selection of compatible bottle/nipple and identify individualized therapeutic positioning, oral feeding techniques, and strategies to support coordination of suck-swallow with breathing. The authors' NICU actively encourages breast feeding as integral to the transition to oral feeding. A dedicated lactation consultant meets with each mother shortly after birth and provides education and assistance to help establish breast milk supply and encourage maintenance with a regular schedule of pumping. As an infant approaches the appropriate gestational age, mothers are encouraged to provide infants with the opportunity to engage in non-nutritive sucking at the breast during Kangaroo Care. Breast feeding opportunities supported by a lactation consultant are offered as part of an infant's individualized feeding plan. Goals of oral feeding in the authors' NICU are consistent adherence to our infant-led philosophy and to each infant's individualized oral feeding plan, and to promote a positive bonding oral feeding experience for both parent and baby.

Although long-awaited and welcome, discharge can often be a stress-inducing time for parents. All team members participate in discharge planning, which includes support for the transition to outpatient care and identification of resources to address uninterrupted continuation of medical care and therapeutic interventions when identified as an immediate need. Referral for longitudinal developmental follow-up is also included.

Meeting Milestones: Developmental/Interprofessional Follow-up for the Premature Infant

Premature infants are widely recognized as at-risk for various neurobehavioral impairments including, but not limited to, cerebral palsy, autism, and attention deficit hyperactivity disorder. Findings also indicate that slightly under half of the population of moderately low and very low birth weight infants are also at risk for demonstration of early abnormal movement patterns and postural instability with later-occurring developmental coordination disorders and minor neurologic dysfunction.[20] Cognitive, neuropsychological, and behavior problems co-occur at a higher prevalence than neuromotor and neurosensory impairment. Performance of preterm infants compared with their full-term peers at preschool age was found to be deficient across the areas of language, attention, memory, visual-motor and visual-spatial processing, and executive functioning.[21,22]

Studies have demonstrated evidence for improved cognitive, behavior, and motor outcomes of premature infants when provided with early educational and therapeutic interventions, making developmental monitoring and early referral for necessary services crucial to support optimal outcomes for these children.[23–25]

The authors' outpatient model for high-risk infant follow-up transitions responsibility for developmental monitoring from the neonatologists to developmental pediatricians. Preterm infants born at 34 weeks or younger are automatically referred for developmental follow-up upon discharge from the authors' NICU. Participants in the infant follow-up program also include infants over 34 weeks with any pre-existing medical or genetic diagnosis that places them at risk of neurodevelopmental deficits.

The team includes developmental pediatricians, physical and occupational therapists, audiologists, speech-language pathologists, and a social worker. Initial evaluation with the developmental pediatrician is scheduled to take place at 4 months corrected age. Additional office visits are scheduled every 6 months over the first 2 years and beyond on an annual basis when continuing developmental monitoring is deemed appropriate. Developmental pediatricians identify undiagnosed or emerging medical/genetic comorbidities; track developmental progress across the domains of gross/fine motor, cognitive/linguistic, and behavior/social interaction; make referrals for necessary therapeutic interventions; and coordinate medical follow-up with each child's pediatrician. It is important to establish strong working relationships with local community pediatricians. As a children's hospital an integrated team of pediatric medical specialists is available to meet infant needs for specialized medical follow-up. The team relies upon community pediatricians to encourage participation in high-risk infant follow-up and to follow through with recommended therapeutic and early intervention services. Parents of premature infants are often exhausted and overwhelmed with the burden of unexpected medical care in the home and juggling of work with other family responsibilities and may not prioritize developmental follow-up until their infant has missed developmental milestones and has fallen behind. It is important for pediatricians to share positive outcome data related to early identification and intervention with parents of their premature patients during office visits.

On a case-by-case basis, outpatient follow-up with a physical or occupational therapist may be initiated immediately following discharge or recommended to take place within 1 to 2 months. Physical therapists play an active role in the surveillance, prevention, and treatment of torticollis and plagiocephaly. Early gross/fine motor assessment includes evaluation of postural control and stability, identification of functional vs aberrant motor patterns, and observation of visual tracking and reach/grasping patterns. Therapeutic intervention is offered to establish functional movement patterns and support attainment of gross/fine motor milestones and development of visual-motor skills.

In adherence with universal hearing screening guidelines, newborn hearing screening is performed prior to discharge from the NICU. Infants with high-risk history, including prematurity with extended NICU stay and medical/genetic diagnoses that are highly associated with hearing loss are referred for ABR testing at 3 months and follow-up of hearing acuity again in the soundfield at the corrected age of 12 months to rule out possibility of any late-onset hearing loss that could negatively impact development of speech and language. Infants identified with hearing loss are followed by both audiologist and pediatric otolaryngologist, provided with any needed medical intervention, fit with hearing aids and assessed for candidacy for cochlear implant when appropriate.

Premature infants with a diagnosed oral feeding and/or swallowing disorder are transitioned from inpatient to outpatient therapy provided by a speech-language pathologist with the requisite education, training, and experience in treating pediatric dysphagia. The subsegment of premature infants who are very low birth weight and present with chronic lung disease or structural or cardiac anomalies are at the most risk for persisting feeding difficulties. Therapeutic intervention is provided to improve effectiveness, efficiency, and coordination of nutritive sucking and help reduce dependence upon alternative nutritional support. Intervention can continue as necessary to address longer-term oral-motor skill development and attainment of age-expected oral feeding transitions (puree → soft textured solids → chewable table food; breast/bottle → cup/straw drinking). Speech-language pathologists also evaluate and provide therapeutic intervention to establish and expand prelinguistic skills, language comprehension, nonverbal and verbal expression, and oral motor skills that support consonant production and functional articulation.

Parent education, participation, and provision of home carryover activities are an integral part of all therapeutic interventions provided across professional disciplines. All team members are knowledgeable with regard to additional available community resources and the referral process for government-funded state-run early intervention services. Consultation with the social worker can be arranged to provide information and guidance with respect to application for government financial resources. Short-term counseling may be provided to support parents and families dealing with competing priorities and the demands of caring for a premature infant at home. Longer-term mental health resources are provided when needed.

SUMMARY

Premature infants currently account for over 9% of all live births. The population of moderately and very low birth weight infants, is at the greatest risk for life-long cognitive, language, neuropsychological, and behavioral deficits. Addressing cultural change in the NICU and embracing a philosophy of developmental care that minimizes the negative effects of stress upon the developing brain and is responsive to the infant's behavior is necessary to improve developmental outcomes. Proactive developmental monitoring (from an interprofessional perspective) following NICU discharge and timely provision of early intervention including therapeutic (PT, OT, and SLT) and educational services are also essential. Parental support to address barriers to participation in early intervention services including issues related to access, financial burden, and psychosocial concerns is needed. It is hypothesized that optimal outcomes for premature infants would best be achieved when developmental care provided while in the NICU is paired with proactive neurodevelopmental follow-up after discharge and timely access to early intervention services of adequate frequency and intensity. Future studies that evaluate infant outcomes given this combined approach are recommended.

REFERENCES

1. Martin JA, Hamilton BE, Osterman MJ, et al. Births: final data for 2015. Natl Vital Stat Rep 2017;66:1.
2. Als H. Toward a syntactive theory of development: promise for the assessment and support of infant individuality. Infant Ment Health J 1982;3:229–43.
3. Als H, Lawhon G, Brown E, et al. Individualized behavioral and environmental care for the very low birth weight preterm infant at high risk for bronchopulmonary dysplasia: neonatal intensive care unit and developmental outcome. Pediatrics 1986;78:1123–32.
4. Anand KJ, Scalzo FM. Can adverse neonatal experiences alter brain development and subsequent behavior? Biol Neonate 2000;77:69–82.
5. Lai MC, Huang LT. Effects of early life stress on neuroendocrine and neurobehavior: mechanisms and implications. Pediatr Neonatol 2011;52:122–9.
6. Als H, Gilkerson L. The role of relationship-based developmentally supportive newborn intensive care in strengthening outcome of preterm infants. Semin Perinatol 1997;21:178–89.
7. Als H, Gilkerson L, Duffy FH, et al. A three-center, randomized, controlled trial of individualized developmental care for very low birth weight preterm infants: medical, neurodevelopmental, parenting, and caregiving effects. J Dev Behav Pediatr 2003;24:399–408.
8. Als H, Duffy FH, McAnulty GB, et al. Early experience alters brain function and structure. Pediatrics 2004;113:846–57.
9. Kleberg A, Westrup B, Stjernqvist K, et al. Indications of improved cognitive development at one year of age among infants born very prematurely who received care based on the Newborn Individualized Developmental Care and Assessment Program (NIDCAP). Early Hum Dev 2002;68:83–91.
10. Westrup B, Bohm B, Lagercrantz H, et al. Preschool outcome in children born very prematurely and cared for according to the Newborn Individualized Developmental Care and Assessment Program (NIDCAP). Acta Paediatr 2004;93:498–507.
11. Als H, Duffy FH, McAnulty GB, et al. Is the Newborn Individualized Developmental Care and Assessment Program (NIDCAP) effective for preterm infants with intrauterine growth restriction? J Perinatol 2011;31:130–6.
12. Als H, Duffy FH, McAnulty G, et al. NIDCAP improves brain function and structure in preterm infants with severe intrauterine growth restriction. J Perinatol 2012;32:797–803.
13. McAnulty G, Duffy FH, Kosta S, et al. School-age effects of the newborn individualized developmental care and assessment program for preterm infants with intrauterine growth restriction: preliminary findings. BMC Pediatr 2013;13:25.
14. Feldman R, Eidelman AI. Skin-to-skin contact (Kangaroo Care) accelerates autonomic and neurobehavioural maturation in preterm infants. Dev Med Child Neurol 2003;45:274–81.

15. Feldman R, Eidelman AI, Sirota L, et al. Comparison of skin-to-skin (kangaroo) and traditional care: parenting outcomes and preterm infant development. Pediatrics 2002;110:16–26.
16. Ohgi S, Fukuda M, Moriuchi H, et al. Comparison of kangaroo care and standard care: behavioral organization, development, and temperament in healthy, low-birth-weight infants through 1 year. J Perinatol 2002;22:374–9.
17. Loewy J, Stewart K, Dassler AM, et al. The effects of music therapy on vital signs, feeding, and sleep in premature infants. Pediatrics 2013;131:902–18.
18. Rodriguez RG, Pattini AE. Neonatal intensive care unit lighting: update and recommendations. Arch Argent Pediatr 2016;114:361–7.
19. Ludwig SM, Waitzman KA. Changing feeding documentation to reflect infant-driven feeding practice. Newborn Infant Nurs Rev 2007;7:155–60.
20. Ferrari F, Gallo C, Pugliese M, et al. Preterm birth and developmental problems in the preschool age. Part I: minor motor problems. J Matern Fetal Neonatal Med 2012;25:2154–9.
21. Arpi E, Ferrari F. Preterm birth and behaviour problems in infants and preschool-age children: a review of the recent literature. Dev Med Child Neurol 2013;55:788–96.
22. Pugliese M, Rossi C, Guidotti I, et al. Preterm birth and developmental problems in infancy and preschool age part II: cognitive, neuropsychological and behavioural outcomes. J Matern Fetal Neonatal Med 2013;26:1653–7.
23. McCormick MC, Brooks-Gunn J, Buka SL, et al. Early intervention in low birth weight premature infants: results at 18 years of age for the Infant Health and Development Program. Pediatrics 2006;117:771–80.
24. Nordhov SM, Ronning JA, Ulvund SE, et al. Early intervention improves behavioral outcomes for preterm infants: randomized controlled trial. Pediatrics 2012;129:e9–16.
25. Spittle A, Treyvaud K. The role of early developmental intervention to influence neurobehavioral outcomes of children born preterm. Semin Perinatol 2016;40:542–8.

Interprofessional Collaborative Practice in Early Intervention

Kathy L. Coufal, PhD[a],*, Juliann J. Woods, PhD[b]

KEYWORDS

- Interprofessional practice and education • Early intervention
- Teaming and collaboration • Family partnerships

KEY POINTS

- Early intervention is an interdisciplinary field with a history of collaborative teamwork that contributes to and benefits from interprofessional collaborative practice.
- Although children with disabilities younger than age 3 and their families are served in multiple settings and service delivery models, interprofessional collaborative practice is the recommended approach to ensure coordination and to maximize family participation.
- The SLP in early intervention provides assessment and intervention services and informational resources supports to the child, family, and other members of the team.
- Competencies clearly delineate the roles and responsibilities of the SLP in EI.
- Engaging families in the intervention process is a linchpin of early intervention that involves the SLP in coaching and consultative services.

This article provides a conceptual framework for speech-language pathologist (SLP) services in early intervention (EI) contexts, including pediatric practices or medical homes, based on the principles of interprofessional collaboration. Specifically, these are identifying key roles and responsibilities of SLPs working as members of interprofessional teams to provide family-centered, culturally responsive services that support children's development in natural contexts and the inclusion of families and other caregivers as essential members of the interprofessional team. The history of collaboration, EI, and the role of SLPs as members of the EI team are summarized. The

Disclosures: Neither author has any financial disclosures to report. Both authors have university affiliations and as such, represent their employers as part of their respective nonfinancial disclosures.
[a] Department of Special Education and Communication Disorders University of Nebraska-Omaha, 6100 Dodge Street, Roskens Hall 512, Omaha, NE 68182, USA; [b] School of Communication Science & Disorders Florida State University, 201 West Bloxham, Warren Building, Tallahassee, FL 32306-1200, USA
* Corresponding author.
E-mail address: kcoufal@unomaha.edu

Pediatr Clin N Am 65 (2018) 143–155
https://doi.org/10.1016/j.pcl.2017.08.027
0031-3955/18/© 2017 Elsevier Inc. All rights reserved.
pediatric.theclinics.com

competencies mandated for interprofessional education and practice are juxtaposed with the principles of highest quality EI and guidelines for SLPs.

INTERPROFESSIONAL COLLABORATIVE PRACTICE DEFINED

Interprofessional collaborative practice is a concept that is currently shared among many disciplines and has grown in acceptance among professional organizations related to all aspects of health care and education (eg,[1,2]). It is not a singular model of services but a process that is grounded in theories and practices that are evidence-based and reflective of a philosophy that is holistic, culturally responsive, and client/family centered. As such, the definitions are aligned with the preprofessional education competencies, professional practice competencies and processes, and the processes and outcomes necessary for effective team work. The following are the operational definitions provided by the Interprofessional Education Collaborative (IPEC). [3(p8)]. As is evident, these are aligned with and grew out of definitions provided by the World Health Organization.[4] It is important to recognize that in defining the competencies for preprofessionals, the intent is to define them in a trajectory for professional practice among disciplines and across services.

OPERATIONAL DEFINITIONS
Interprofessional Education

"When students from two or more professions learn about, from and with each other to enable effective collaboration and improve health outcomes."[4]

Interprofessional Collaborative Practice

"When multiple health workers from different professional backgrounds work together with patients, families, [Caregivers], and communities to deliver the highest quality of care."[4]

Interprofessional Teamwork

The levels of cooperation, coordination, and collaboration characterizing the relationships between professions in delivering person-centered care.

Interprofessional Team-Based Care

Care delivered by intentionally created, usually small work groups in health care or education who are recognized by others and by themselves as having a collective identity and shared responsibility for a patient or student, or group of patients or students (eg, primary care team, student support team, and individualized family support plan team).

IS THIS NEW?

The interest in collaborative practice has a long-standing history and scholarly activity that includes nearly all special service professions, as summarized by Gutkin.[5] The concept of collaborative service delivery derived from processes first attributed to work in the areas of community counseling,[6] and later applied to educational settings, evolving from the metal health literature.[7,8] Coufal[9] summarized the critical competencies essential to the collaborative planning and problem-solving model as emphasizing communication skills; mutual respect; ecological and holistic assessment and intervention; and assessment of the team's accountability, processes, and outcomes. These characteristics are essential to interprofessional collaborative processes, regardless of the persons being served or the professional disciplines represented within a team. The medical home process and Individuals With Disabilities Education Act (IDEA) Part C policy also support nurturing relationships and family-centered care for families and interprofessional education for the pediatric team.[10]

WHAT HISTORICALLY HAS BEEN DISCUSSED IN THE LITERATURE FOR SPEECH-LANGUAGE PATHOLOGY?

Working as a member of an interprofessional team is an IDEA-legislated requirement[11] and a recommended practice to address the diverse needs of young children eligible for EI and their families.[2,12] Challenges, such as fragmentation of services, lack of coordination in types and frequency of service provision, contradictory intervention approaches, lack of communication, and limited collaboration among team members, are frequently identified by families and described in literature related to teaming practices.[13,14] Children at risk for or with delays and disabilities and their families require services and support from a variety of professionals aligned with the educational, social, and health care sectors in the community. Shifting from a "discipline centered" approach to a model that focuses on joint decision-making and shared responsibility among those involved with providing services draws attention to the competencies needed for SLPs as members of an interprofessional team. The call for interprofessional collaboration is not new to SLPs, but is currently receiving greater emphasis from health care providers.

More than 25 years ago, Coufal[15] and others published a collection of articles focused on the need for and processes of collaborative service delivery, targeting SLPs working with young children and families. Implementation examples of assessment and continuity of care for infants and their families were provided by Crais[16] and Laadt-Bruno and coworkers.[17] Furthermore, Rowan and coworkers[18] documented an interdisciplinary infancy specialization program that prepared preservice students from four disciplines in the best practices for using a multidisciplinary collaborative team approach to EI.

In 2004, the IDEA was reauthorized with further emphasis on the importance of enhancing the capacity of families to meet their child's needs. EI, as defined in Part C of IDEA, continued to support family-centered, multidisciplinary approaches in natural environments rather than child-focused direct intervention. Accordingly, the American Speech-Language-Hearing Association (ASHA)[1] identified roles and responsibilities for SLPs working in EI. Services must be (1) family-centered, culturally and linguistically responsive; (2) supporting development and fostering children's participation in daily routines and natural environments; and (3) comprehensive, coordinated, team-based services that are based on the highest quality of evidence available. "Of particular note is that intervention be focused on adult caregivers of the child, while including everyday routines, activities, places, and people into sessions. This necessitates preparation of professionals across disciplines to provide services in natural environments, which includes not only where the services are provided but also all elements of what the services encompass, who provides services and the roles and responsibilities of the team members."[19(pp177–178)]

Consistent with the ASHA Council on Academic Accreditation guidelines for graduate programs and the Council for Clinical Certification, students must demonstrate knowledge and skill competencies that prepare them to work with individuals across the lifespan. Therefore, it is incumbent on graduate programs to include performance criteria for master's degree students that include key content and skills relevant to the EI population. The ASHA 2012 Health Care Landscape Summit included participants representing 70 health care administrators, clinical directors, clinicians, researchers, academicians, consultants, and consumer groups. Interprofessional education was identified as one of several top priorities as reimbursement and patient care models shift away from fee-for-service to pay-for-performance and value-based service delivery. Key elements of interprofessional education were determined to include specific courses in graduate schools, opportunities for collaborative clinical education and practicum experiences, and collaborative practice in health care settings to maximize patients' functional outcomes.[20]

Despite this history, a national survey of universities providing graduate degrees in communication sciences and disorders revealed limited exposure for students to curricular content and clinical practica that focused on the knowledge and skills necessary for professionals working in EI settings.[19] It is clear that preprofessional education and professional development must continue to provide opportunities to develop knowledge and skills in the context of interprofessional education and clinical practice.

Guralnick and Bruder[21] recently summarized the literature of evidence-based practices in four key areas that defined goals of early childhood programs over the past 40 years: (1) access, (2) accommodations and feasibility, (3) developmental progress, and (4) social integration. In particular, they discuss recommendations that emphasize personnel preparation, accreditation and licensing, and team processes. Their findings and recommendations note that preservice programs generally are discipline-specific, as are the personnel standards that guide the accreditation of higher education programs and the states' licensure requirements. They note there is lack of congruence among the various agencies and the competencies needed to provide best practices are not consistent with national standards and goals, derived from evidence-based practices. Their recommendations call for congruence among higher education programs, state policies for certification, and national organizations' prescribed competencies among all disciplines preparing professionals to provide EI services. "Only then will the United States be able to demonstrate the availability of a quality workforce that is able to effectively and collaboratively implement curricular and instructional modifications, adaptations, and instructional practices to benefit all children..."[(p173)] With nearly 100,000 members of ASHA[22] reporting they work with EI populations, the importance of personnel preparation is paramount.

WHAT IS KNOWN ABOUT SPEECH-LANGUAGE PATHOLOGY IN EARLY INTERVENTION?

As one member of an EI interprofessional team, SLPs play an important role in helping shape a child's future. Depending on the child's immediate needs and the concerns of the family and other professionals, the SLP participates in a variety of roles that may range from being the primary EI service provider, to providing consultation to the family or other professionals who have a larger role with the child, coaching caregivers, or joining in classroom interventions. Each of these roles requires competence in the discipline and as a team member and partner working in unison with the family. SLPs often play a key role in working with children who have needs in the areas of communication, language, speech, feeding and swallowing, cognition, hearing, emergent literacy, autism spectrum disorder, and social/emotional behavior. SLPs also play a critical role in the assessment and provision of assistive technologies, including the use of augmentative and alternative communication. Within EI, the SLP must continually assess current and future communication needs, partnering with families and other discipline-specific professionals to promote and support present and ongoing developmental change for the child, family, and prospective social, behavioral, and adaptive functions.

In EI, SLPs are expected to do the following:

- Understand typical development across domains from birth to age 3;
- Describe developmental delays/disorders in young children;
- Explain the impact of communication delays and disorders in speech, language, hearing, emergent literacy, and swallowing/feeding, on development;
- Identify the genetic, biologic, and environmental risk factors associated with communication disorders;
- Have a theoretic and evidence-based background for eliciting communication;
- Have the skills that support family interactions that consider cultural beliefs, values, and priorities for their child; and
- Have knowledge of federal and state laws and policies that pertain to EI.

SLPs work in a range of job settings and across differing types of interprofessional teams. In settings where SLPs are part of an interprofessional team, their contributions may vary depending on the knowledge and skills they possess and those represented by other professionals on the team. For example, an SLP who has expertise in feeding/swallowing may be on an EI team with an Occupational Therapist (OT) who also has feeding/swallowing expertise. The team would collectively decide how to handle the overlap in expertise held by the OT and SLP. The end result may be that the SLP would provide feeding/swallowing services to children in one geographic region or may work exclusively with children who have primary speech and language issues that match the SLP's other areas of expertise. It is important also that the family's input on service delivery and participation in be considered.

Regardless of setting or service delivery option, EI services and supports are based on the same core principles.[2,23,24] The first principle, that services and supports are family centered and culturally responsive, emphasizes the unique role of the family and their beliefs, values, priorities, and preferences in the development and implementation of an individualized plan for the child. Families are active participants and decision makers throughout the process, integrating their cultural and linguistic values and practices. Developmentally supportive services that promote children's participation in their natural environments is the second principle. Based on theoretic and empirical models of child development, acquisition and use of communication that occurs within a social and cultural framework is the target. Services and supports offer realistic and authentic learning experiences and promote meaningful and functional communication with family members, peers, caregivers, and team members. The third principle, that services are comprehensive, coordinated, and team-based, speaks to the essence of how SLPs deliver services as one of several professionals working with the child and family. Communication and collaboration to ensure the child and family priorities are addressed efficiently and effectively is the responsibility of every team member regardless of the method of service delivery. Finally, services and supports are based on the highest quality internal and external evidence that is available. The integration of the highest quality and most recent empirical research, informed professional judgment and expertise, and family preferences and values guides the service delivery model identified for the child and the manner in which the roles of the SLP are enacted.

The move from a culture of discipline-specific education and EI services for families necessitates an inclusionary team approach in which every member develops and uses strong relational skills to effectively coordinate their work with other members of the team. In professional education programs, preparing SLPs to be successful in EI requires that graduate programs create diverse learning environments that engage students in developing their understanding of how their discipline-specific knowledge is integral to team-based decision making. To that end, faculty and clinical educators must engage with "colleagues across disciplines and immerse students in learning opportunities that engage critical thinking and effective communication about roles, responsibilities, team processes, leadership, and systems theory. We cannot presume that students will infer such knowledge or develop effective interpersonal, team-based skills unless they have overt instruction, models, and meaningful experiences in which to be engaged, followed by feedback from more experienced professionals."[25] Preparing future professionals and those SLPs working in EI must embrace, model, and demonstrate that services are defined by and delivered from the framework of the IPEC principles, wedded with the core principles of EI and the roles and responsibilities of SLPs.

- The guiding principles of IPEC intersect with the interprofessional collaborative team approach to promote high-quality EI service provision.
- The four core competencies defined by IPEC[3] mirror the guiding principles of early childhood education and intervention.
- The recent updates to the IPEC report (2016) more explicitly embed the four core competencies and subcompetencies under the single domain of Interprofessional Collaborative practice. "Instead of depicting four domains within interprofessional collaborative practice (values/ethics, roles/responsibilities, interprofessional communication, teams and teamwork), the four topical areas fall under the single domain of interprofessional collaboration in which four core competencies and related sub-competencies now reside."[(p9)] These core competencies define the goals and outcomes for both preprofessional preparation and professional practices across disciplines. The intent is to frame the perspective for all disciplines to provide services that are "community and population oriented, and patient and family-centered."[(p9)]

Competency 1

Work with individuals of other professions to maintain a climate of mutual respect and shared values (Values/Ethics for Interprofessional Practice).

Competency 2

Use the knowledge of one's own role and those of other professions to appropriately assess and address the health care needs of patients and to promote and advance the health of populations (Roles/Responsibilities).

Competency 3

Communicate with patients, families, communities, and professionals in health and other fields in a responsive and responsible manner that supports a team approach to the promotion and maintenance of health and the prevention and treatment of disease (Interprofessional Communication).

Competency 4

Apply relationship-building values and the principles of team dynamics to perform effectively in different team roles to plan, deliver, and evaluate patient/population-centered care and population health programs and policies that are safe, timely, efficient, effective, and equitable (Teams and Teamwork). Develop family-centered services and supports that are culturally and linguistically responsive.

IMPLICATIONS FOR SPEECH-LANGUAGE PATHOLOGY IN EARLY INTERVENTION
Interprofessional Education Collaborative Competency 1: Values/Ethics for Interprofessional Practice/Early Intervention Principle 3: Comprehensive, Team-Based, and Coordinated

- Values and Ethics: all members of a team embrace and use those qualities of good team membership in a comprehensive approach that is inclusive, sensitive, responsive, and embedded in natural contexts. That teams maintain a climate of mutual respect and shared values. The SLP needs to be sensitive to unique cultural and linguistic differences among families and can contribute to team members' collective understanding of how these impact all aspects of service delivery.

Related Speech-Language Pathology Competencies for Early Intervention

- Interact with caregivers using communication that is matched to the adult and tuned to the developmental level of the child
- Develop family-centered services and supports that are culturally and linguistically responsive
- Integrate expertise of team members across developmental areas to ensure comprehensive assessment and intervention
- Embed functional intervention outcomes in everyday routines in natural environments
- Understand the impact of developmental communication delays and disorders on families and children
- Reflect the role of cultural beliefs, values, and priorities for the child, family, and service providers, including cultural influences on communication and social interactions in practice
- Be knowledgeable of federal and state laws, policies, and procedures pertaining to services (including transition services) for infants and toddlers with, or at risk for, disabilities

Interprofessional Education Collaborative Competency 2: Roles/Responsibilities/Early Intervention Principle 4: High-Quality and Best Evidence

- Roles and Responsibilities for Collaborative Practice: The second IPEC core competency relates to eight specific responsibilities that are defined within the scope of practice for SLPs.[26] Students preparing for entry into the profession must demonstrate the foundational knowledge and skills as relate to human function: psychological, physical, social, cultural, linguistic, cognitive, and biologic. These roles are common to all professions. The task is to bring the unique knowledge of human communication together with that of other professions. The SLP must use knowledge of one's own role and those of other professionals to address the needs of the population served.

Related Speech-Language Pathology Competencies for Early Intervention

Prevention

- Knowledge of appropriate prevention, wellness, and health-promotion activities
- Apply strategies for monitoring children's development and family concerns
- Select appropriate prevention activities for varying contexts and situations
- Adapt prevention activities and methods in accord with cultural and linguistic characteristics of the child and family

Screening evaluation and assessment

- Derive screening, evaluation, and assessment data from multiple sources (including parent report) and using multiple methods
- Knowledge of roles of interdisciplinary and transdisciplinary team procedures in the evaluation, diagnosis, and assessment for infants and toddlers with developmental delays and disabilities
- Knowledge of options and strategies for involvement of paraprofessionals, interpreters, and other team members and support personnel in the screening, assessment, and evaluation process
- Observe, document, and interpret child behaviors across appropriate natural environments and within typical routines and activities
- Document and integrate concerns, priorities, and observations from families, caregivers, and other professionals in the evaluation and assessment process

Planning and implementing intervention

- Communicate effectively with family, caregivers, and other team members regarding strengths, needs, program development, and monitoring
- Facilitate collaborative problem solving with families, caregivers, and other team members to deliver and monitor interventions
- Teach families, caregivers, or other professionals specific intervention strategies as appropriate
- Communicate about service delivery models to meet the needs of the individual child and family (eg, direct service, collaborative consultation, playgroup-based, parent coaching)

Consultation with and education of the team and families

- Through consultation and education with caregivers and other team members, promote the implementation of strategies targeting the child's development of communication
- Provide coaching and indirect services, when appropriate, through consultation that supports caregivers and other professionals in the use of indirect communication stimulation
- Promote communication development in natural contexts
- Provide ongoing monitoring, consultation, and participation in intervention plans and program updates

Engage in service coordination

- Appropriately work with the mandated service coordination processes, as defined by IDEA, Part C

Support the child's transition to other services and programs

- Provide input to transition plans, as appropriate
- Support the seamless transition of children and families as changes in programs/placements occur

Advocacy

- Promote awareness and public support for EI through participation in education, policy development, and dissemination of information to a broad audience

Advancement of knowledge base

- As an active consumer of professional literature and through ongoing professional development, continue to expand the use of research through evidence-based practices
- Advance the knowledge base in EI and communication sciences and disorders through participation in research and demonstration projects

Interprofessional Education Collaborative Competency 3: Interprofessional Communication/Early Intervention Principle 2: Family-Centered and Culturally Responsive

Interprofessional communication

The third core competency states that all members of the team communicate with clients, families, communities and other professionals in a responsive manner that supports a team approach. To develop an effective team requires dynamic, open communication among all members. Teams evolve—they work to become more effective. The SLP, like other members of the team, must communicate evidence in a jargon-free, case-relevant manner. The SLP who can effectively explain how evidence from research relates to the family and child of concern is a positive contributor to the assessment and treatment objectives. This requires disclosure and transparency among team members to build trust in our ability and that of others to fulfill professional roles.

- Use evidence-based communication strategies to facilitate family-centered discussions that encourage family participation and decision-making
- Work to effectively coordinate services and supports with other team members
- Develop goals based on family priorities and shared across team members
- Engage in open, dynamic and regular communication based on commitment to the family and mutual regard and trust

Interprofessional Education Collaborative Competency 4: Teams and Teamwork/Early Intervention Principle 1: Family-Centered and Culturally Responsive

The fourth core competency requires collaborative planning and problem solving that is systematic, ongoing, and frequently evaluated as to the effectiveness of the team. When caregivers are active members of the team processes, they become more proficient in their ability to contribute to decision-making and are more engaged in fulfilling their role as primary interventionists for their child. Preprofessional education and clinical practica need to provide the foundations necessary for students from all disciplines to develop their skills in team-based care. By immersing students in interprofessional learning contexts, they develop the underlying foundations and the applied skills necessary to function as effective members of an interprofessional team.

- Apply relationship building values and principles of team dynamics to perform different team roles that deliver patient-centered care
- Engage all team members in collaborative planning and problem solving
- Use team process to derive mutual goals and interventions with shared accountability
- Promote team development, shared knowledge, and teach others the skills of collaborative planning and problem solving

Related Speech-Language Pathology Competencies for Early Intervention

- Collaborative design of intervention services to achieve mutually defined target outcomes

- Implementing strategies to function as an effective member of an interprofessional programming team
- Establishing a collaborative, supportive relationship with families
- Integrating information about the child from multiple sources into an integrated developmental summary
- Developing functional outcomes that help the child and family to be successful and included within his or her natural environment
- Helping families develop their advocacy and problem-solving skills

FAMILY PARTNERSHIPS ON THE TEAM

The collaborative process between the family, the SLP, and other team members is integral to the assessment, planning, and intervention processes. Experiences with and expectations for communication are grounded in the sociocultural ecology of the family. Learning from the children's caregivers about communication in their everyday settings provides the context for the child's profile[13,27] and actively engages family members in the decision-making process for their children's intervention.

Several intervention studies and systematic reviews have shown that parents and other caregivers can effectively use communication strategies and supports with positive effects on their children's communication outcomes (eg, see Refs.[28–30]). The interventions examined in these studies were based on the established framework that parents can and do have an instrumental role in their children's communication and language development[31,32] and teaching parents and other caregivers to use specific communication interactions and support strategies can enhance their children's skills.

When examining parent-implemented intervention studies for EI, two additional considerations related to interprofessional collaboration and IDEA Part C service delivery are noted: the service location and the parent's role. IDEA Part C stipulates that EI services and supports are designed to build the families' capacity to support their children's development and are to be provided in their natural environments, including physical locations (ie, setting) and the family's routines and activities (ie, context).[11,24] This means that EI service providers must be competent to conduct home visits and to consult with teachers and child care providers in community early care and education programs rather than conduct services in clinical or medical-based facilities. In addition, the interventions are to be embedded where and when the child participates in routines, such as during mealtime, play, or washing hands. The SLP must be able to learn from the parents what their priorities are for their child and which routines and activities are the best contextual match for the parent to support the child's learning.

Family capacity-building underscores an important distinction among the broad category of parent-implemented interventions. Although the terms "training" and "coaching" are often used interchangeably or in a nonspecific manner, there are important differences between the two approaches[33] and important implications for interprofessional education and collaboration. Specifically, training parents to implement intervention in predetermined intervention contexts (eg, child care, clinic setting) is different than collaborating with parents as decision makers in the process of coaching them to embed intervention in their everyday routines. Parent training often entails the SLP providing information, modeling strategies while the parent watches, and providing specific instructions to the parents on what and how to use strategies within play activities (eg, see Ref.[28]). However, coaching parents in a manner congruent with family capacity building principles includes parents as active participants, integral decision makers, and collaborators in how, where, and when the intervention is implemented.[30,34,35] Interventions using a parent coaching approach focus on the triadic interaction of the interventionist supporting the bidirectional parent-child interactions and communication.[27,36] Therefore, the SLP must be able to engage in interactions that support the communication between the parent and child, and be able to identify and build on the intervention strategies the parent is using effectively while problem solving with the parent on additional strategies and contexts that can expand the child's communication repertoire. To be determined as effective and efficient, parent-implemented communication interventions for young children overall should address the needs of the child and of the parent, increasing the knowledge and skills required of the interprofessional team. Competencies necessary for coaching parents to embed interventions throughout their daily interactions and routines are congruent with those identified (eg, respectful and responsive interactions, application of evidence-based practices, collaborative communication, problem solving and planning). SLPs who coach parents must first recognize the diversity of potential relationships between parents and professionals and be aware of their own cultural values and expectations while simultaneously understanding their role to support the essential relationship between each parent and child. The following competencies are important additions for coaching in EI.

Related Speech-Language Pathology Competencies for Coaching

- Use knowledge about parent's priorities, preferences, and culture to inform coaching practices ("contextual" fit) and build consensus on developmental goals
- Identify family strengths as a foundation for building their capacity to learn and use new strategies and routines throughout their day (start where they are) that embed practice on communication goals
- Observe family members interacting with their child in meaningful routines, coach them to embed interventions, and provide feedback to them in multiple contexts to promote generalization
- Encourage caregiver reflection and problem solving on what worked and what other outcomes, strategies, and routines to practice throughout the day

SUMMARY AND DISCUSSION

The sheer numbers of children receiving EI, the importance of the services relative to children's later academic success, and the importance of service coordination to support family participation and satisfaction elevates the importance of interprofessional education and practice. With more than 100,000 SLPs reported to be working in EI and the continued call for greater numbers of graduates prepared to assume roles on EI teams, the call for action is great. It calls for continuing emphasis on comprehensive, coordinated education and ongoing professional development to promote the necessary knowledge and skills required of individuals and teams serving the youngest clients and their families. It is not sufficient to simply assign professionals from diverse disciplines to be team members. It is essential that every member of the team embrace the underlying principles, engage in personal and team reflection on the efficacy of the program for the child and family, and the assessment of team functioning as a whole and for each member's contribution to the process. Only through dynamic processes and continuous quality improvement will teams derive the highest quality of service provision and truly model the critical principles of interprofessional collaboration.

REFERENCES

1. American Speech-Language-Hearing Association. Roles and responsibilities of speech-language pathologists in early intervention: guidelines [Guidelines]. 2008. Available at: www.asha.org/policy. Accessed April 26, 2017.
2. Division for Early Childhood. DEC Recommended Practices in Early Intervention/Early Childhood Special Education. 2014. Available at: http://www.dec-sped.org/recommended practices. Accessed March 29, 2017.
3. Interprofessional Education Collaborative. Core competencies for interprofessional collaborative practice: 2016 update. Washington, DC: Interprofessional Education Collaborative; 2016.
4. World Health Organization. Framework for action on interprofessional education and collaborative practice. Geneva (Switzerland): Author; 2010. Available at: http://whqlibdoc.who.int/hq/2010/WHO_HRH_HPN_10.3_eng.pdf.
5. Gutkin TB. Conducting consultation research. San Francisco (CA): Jossey-Bass; 1993.
6. Tharp RG, Wetzel RJ. Behavior modification in the natural environment. New York: Academic Press; 1969.
7. Caplan G. Principles of preventive psychiatry. Oxford (England): Basic Books; 1964.
8. Will MC. Educating children with learning problems: a shared responsibility. Except Child 1986;52(5):411–5.
9. Coufal KL. Collaborative consultation for speech-language pathologists. Top Lang Disord 1993;14(1):1–14.
10. Adams RC, Tapia C. Early intervention, IDEA Part C services, and the medical home: collaboration for best practice and best outcomes. Pediatrics 2013; 132(4):e1073–88.
11. Individuals with Disabilities Education Act, 20 U.S.C. § 1400. 2004.
12. ASHA. 2008.
13. Crais E, Woods J. Role of the speech language pathologist in early childhood special education. In: Odom S, Boyd B, Reichow R, et al, editors. Handbook of early childhood special education. Baltimore (MD): Paul H. Brookes Publishing; 2016. p. 363–83.
14. Marturana E, McComish C, Woods JJ, et al. Early intervention teaming and the primary service provider approach: who does what, when, why, and how? Perspect Lang Learn Educ 2011;18:47–52.
15. Coufal KL. Collaborative consultation: a problem-solving process. Top Lang Disord 1993;14(1):vi–vii.
16. Crais ER. Families and professionals as collaborators in assessment. Top Lang Disord 1993;14(1):29–40.
17. Laadt-Bruno G, Lilley PK, Westby C. A collaborative approach to developmental care continuity with infants born at risk and their families. Top Lang Disord 1993; 14(1):15–28.
18. Rowan LE, McCollum JA, Thorp EK. Collaborative graduate education of future early interventionists. Top Lang Disord 1993;14(1):72–80.
19. Francois JR, Coufal KL, Subramanian A. Student preparation for professional practice in early intervention. Commun Disord Q 2015;36(3):177–86.
20. McNeilly L. Health care summit identified need for interprofessional education clinicians, researchers and administrators agree: changes in health care delivery and reimbursement models make interprofessional education and practice a must. Here's what ASHA is doing about it. ASHA Leader 2013;18(6). online-only.

21. Guralnick MJ, Bruder MB. Early childhood inclusion in the United States: goals, current status, and future directions. Infants Young Child 2016;29(3):166–77.
22. American Speech-Language-Hearing Association. Workforce reports. 2013. Available at: http://www.asha.org/research/WorkforceReports/. Accessed April 1, 2017.
23. American Speech-Language-Hearing Association. Core knowledge and skills in early intervention speech-language pathology practice. 2008. Available at: www.asha.org/policy. Accessed April 26, 2017.
24. National Early Childhood Technical Assistance Center. 2008. Workgroup on Principles and Practices in Natural Environments (2008, February). Agreed upon practices for providing early intervention services in natural environments. OSEP TA Community of Practice-Part C Settings.
25. Coufal KL, Scherz J. Interprofessional education in communication sciences and disorders. Access Academics and Research. 2013. Available at: www.asha.org/enews/accessacademics.html. Accessed April 1, 2017.
26. American Speech-Language-Hearing Association. Scope of practice in speech-language pathology. 2007. Available at: www.asha.org/policy. Accessed April 26, 2017.
27. Woods J, Wilcox MJ, Friedman M, et al. Collaborative consultation in natural environments: strategies to enhance family centered supports and services. Lang Speech Hear Serv Sch 2011;42:379–92.
28. Girolametto L, Weitzman E, Clements-Baartman J. Vocabulary intervention for children with Down syndrome: parent training using focused stimulation, infant-toddler intervention. Transdisciplinary J 1998;8(2):109–25.
29. Kaiser AP, Roberts MY. Parent-implemented enhanced milieu teaching with preschool children who have intellectual disabilities. J Speech Lang Hear Res 2013; 56:295–309.
30. Wetherby A, Woods JJ. Effectiveness of early intervention for children with autism spectrum disorders beginning in the second year of life. Top Early Child Spec Education 2006;26(2):67–82.
31. Hart B, Risley TR. Meaningful differences in the everyday experience of young American children. Baltimore (MD): Paul H Brookes Publishing; 1995.
32. Landry SH, Smith KE, Swank PR. Responsive parenting: establishing early foundations for social, communication, and independent problem-solving skills. Dev Psychol 2006;42(4):627–42.
33. Kemp P, Turnbull AP. Coaching with parents in early intervention: an interdisciplinary research synthesis. Infants Young Child 2014;27(4):305–24.
34. Brown JA, Woods JJ. Effects of a triadic parent implemented home based communication intervention for toddlers. J Early Intervention 2015;37(1):44–68.
35. Woods J, Kashinath S, Goldstein H. Effects of embedding caregiver-implemented teaching strategies in daily routines on children's communication outcomes. J Early Intervention 2004;26(3):175–93.
36. Salisbury CL, Cushing LS. Comparison of triadic and provider-led intervention practices in early intervention home visits. Infants Young Child 2013;26(1):28–41.

The Role of the Speech-Language Pathologist in Creating a Model for Interprofessional Practice in an Ambulatory Care Clinic

 CrossMark

Tommie L. Robinson Jr, PhD, CCC-SLP*,
Debra Anderson, MS, CCC-SLP, Sahira Long, MD, IBCLC, FABM

KEYWORDS

- Interprofessional practice • Interprofessional education • Ambulatory services
- Speech-language pathology • Community pediatrics services

KEY POINTS

- There are barriers to accessing speech-language and hearing services in urban settings.
- Collaboration and increased communication among pediatric health care providers is critical to identifying and managing communication disorders in children.
- An interprofessional model for service delivery enhances the care of children with communication disorders and reduces medical errors.

CASE PRESENTATION

Z. Johnson is a 5-year-old African American female patient of the Children's Health Center at Anacostia location (CHC-Anacostia).[1,2] She was born after an uncomplicated pregnancy at 40 weeks gestation. Her neonatal period was complicated by a concern for neonatal sepsis that was treated with a 7-day course of ampicillin and gentamicin. She passed her newborn hearing screen and developed normally through her first year of life with a normal Ages and Stages Questionnaire (ASQ) completed by her parents when she was 9 months of age. Her parents raised a concern about her language development when they brought her to her 15-month well-child care visit

Children's National Health System, Children's Hearing and Speech Center, 111 Michigan Avenue, NW, Washington, DC 20010, USA
* Corresponding author.
E-mail address: trobinso@childrensnational.org

Pediatr Clin N Am 65 (2018) 157–170
https://doi.org/10.1016/j.pcl.2017.08.028
0031-3955/18/© 2017 Elsevier Inc. All rights reserved.

at the age of 16 months. At that time, she was thought to not talk as much as her age-matched family members and only said one word aside from "mommy" and "daddy," albeit inconsistently. An ASQ completed at that time revealed scores below the cutoff in the following domains: communication, fine motor, and problem-solving. Her pediatrician provided a list of activities to promote fine motor and problem-solving development and referred her to the Early Intervention Program (EIP) for evaluation of language. If deemed ineligible for services through the EIP, she was to be referred to the Children's Hearing and Speech Center to begin therapy. Approximately six weeks later she was seen for an emergency room follow-up visit. At that time, her parents reported that she had been evaluated by the EIP and had started receiving speech therapy on a weekly basis, although no documentation from the EIP had been received to confirm this. Per her parents, the EIP recommended a repeat hearing test, so a referral was placed to the Children's Hearing and Speech Center for an audiology evaluation. One month later, at her 18-month well-child care visit, her parents had not yet made an appointment to have her hearing tested and reported that she was on a wait list for a developmental daycare where she could receive services. Per her parents, the EIP was supposed to increase her speech-language therapy to twice weekly for 1-hour sessions; however, all services had been placed on hold pending an insurance transition and awaiting the EIP hiring of a permanent speech-language pathologist (SLP). At that time, she had no words other than "Dada," "Ma," and "Bye." She passed a Modified Checklist for Autism in Toddlers (M-CHAT) screening with two failed items, one of which was critical. In addition, a repeat ASQ demonstrated communication scores below the cutoff with all other areas within normal limits. At her 2-year well-child care visit, she spoke fewer than twenty words and was not combining words but again passed an M-CHAT screen. She was re-referred for an audiology evaluation because this appointment had still not been scheduled. By her 30-month well-child care visit, her parents reported that her speech and language skills were improving with the provision of speech therapy; however, ASQ screening revealed scores below the cutoff in the following domains: communication, gross motor, and problem-solving. She continued to receive speech and occupational therapy through the EIP until she transitioned from a developmental daycare to preschool where an individualized education program (IEP) was developed to provide speech-language and occupational therapy. At the age of 4 years, her school no longer deemed her eligible to receive IEP services and she successfully passed a pure tone hearing screening at her pediatrician's office.

INTRODUCTION

Z. Johnson's case is an example of why interprofessional practice is important for the clinical well-being of patients, especially those in pediatrics. Many of the issues identified in her case could have been avoided, if the team members were part of an interprofessional practice.

Ambulatory care clinics (ACCs) in urban settings are often faced with the stigma of not offering coordinated care for the patients and families that are seen in such care centers. What critics fail to realize and understand is there are many parameters that affect service delivery to patients in urban settings. Factors may include but are not limited to the following:

- Transportation: The inability of the patient to get to services because of transportation challenges related to cost, timing, and availability. Although the two closest Children's National Health System locations where hearing and speech services are offered (Northwest, District of Columbia [DC] and Upper Marlboro, Maryland) are only 8 and 10 miles away, respectively, from the CHC-Anacostia, patients are often reliant on the public transportation system. As such, travel to these two locations can take 45 minutes or 1.5 hours in one direction, respectively. Because most families request appointments at the Northwest DC location, there are often extended wait times for the first available visit. Given these access barriers, children with suspected speech and language delays are often referred to the EIP for speech-language evaluations.

- Lack of education: The parents may not know about the available services or the impact that the service has on the overall wellbeing of the patient. This also stems from the fact that some of the parents are young, inexperienced, and lack knowledge of the typical developmental processes. Often, the parents did not finish high school or required specialized education services to do so.
- Childcare: Families may have more than one child and, in some cases, have more than one child with special needs. It is so easy for clinicians to lose sight of the fact that these families might have several issues with which they are dealing simultaneously. They might not be able to keep an appointment because one child is sick and there is no one to keep him or her in order for the parent to bring the patient to services.
- Inability to pay for services: There are many families who have no insurance or government support to pay for services. These are families who pay out of pocket for medical services. Therefore, if a follow-up visit is a recommendation but the concern is not considered life-threatening, then it may not be a priority among other competing financial obligations.
- Psychosocial challenges: These challenges are personal and social situations that interfere with and take precedence over the need to do follow-up for services. These may include toxic stressors such as neighborhood violence, alcoholism, drug use, employment (or lack thereof), gambling, and involvement with the criminal justice system.
- Personnel factors: The staff from the Division of General Pediatrics and Community Health has limited to no interactions with the staff from the Division of Hearing and Speech. As such, there is a need to develop working relationships between the staff to ensure collaborative success in the joint management of shared patients.

Although these factors play a role in the service delivery process, they are by no means meant as a stereotype for parents of patients seen in ACCs. The point is that there are a lot of issues that affect the lives of individuals in lower socioeconomic areas. Those issues carry over to the ACC, so when referrals are made for speech-language services, the SLP has to take these issues under consideration as well.

A new national report reviews the prevalence and implications for speech-language disorders in children living in poverty and concludes that speech and language disorders affect between 3% and 16% of US children.[1,2] The report further indicates the following:

- More research is needed on the epidemiology of speech and language disorders to enhance understanding of the prevalence, variability by race, ethnicity, and socioeconomic factors.
- Of children with speech and language disorders, 26% live in poor or low-income households; 21% of children who did not present with speech and language disorders live in poverty.
- Children in low-income families are more likely than the general population to exhibit disabilities, including speech and language disorders. Of the 0.31% of

children living in the United States who receive Supplemental Security Income (SSI) benefits for speech and language disorders, 16% were receiving them for a primary speech and language impairment.

- About 40% of SSI children with severe speech and language disorders had other conditions, including intellectual disability, autism spectrum disorder, attention deficit hyperactive disorders, and other neurodevelopmental and behavioral disorders.

There might be several reasons for the increase in percentage rate of children who are in need of services:

- Lack of exposure to language stimulation resources: Parents need to be educated on how to create a language-enriched environment and verbally stimulate their children. Although there is an increase in the use of screens at a younger age with the advent of tablets and digital devices, these items should not be used to replace verbal stimulation activities such as reading, conversation, oral problem-solving, questions, and other forms of human interactions.
- Parents do not have the knowledge and education base: The high school graduation rate in Washington, DC, is 69%. The national graduation rate has hit an all-time high of more than 82% in the 2013 to 2014 school year according to the US Department of Education.[3] As such, the District's graduation rates lag behind the national average.
- Literacy deficit: It is no secret that literacy is the basis for speech and language learning. Evidence indicates that there is a discernible difference in the language skills of children from low-income families when compared with children who are more privileged. The word gap is astounding. In one year, children from low-income families are exposed to 250,000 utterances, whereas their wealthier counter parts are exposed to 4 million.[4] There could be several reasons for this literacy deficit, including that some parents do not know how to facilitate language and literacy and the importance that it plays in life. Other causes may include
  - Limited time or resources to devote to reading to their children
  - Focused communication on necessities, such as what to eat, what to do, and other practical topics
  - Lack of exposure to explore things that are connected to reading
  - Making the mistake of thinking that the role of facilitating language and literacy is the responsibility of teacher
- Parental reporting level is higher: It is possible that the number of individuals requiring speech-language services has increased because more families have realized there can often be a financial benefit through SSI when there is documentation that the child has a disability. The funding would serve to assist the family in meeting very basic needs and can sometimes be the difference in food on the table in a warm environment versus hunger and homelessness.

Although the possible links to the cause of the increase in communication disorders has been explored, there are several overarching factors that affect the lives of the patients in this area that cannot be ignored:

- Encouragement and confidence levels of the parents: These are two important factors that parents must have when raising children. Encouragement is important because it lends the hope and support that are needed in the everyday process of parenting. Parents need to be encouraged, especially when there is a child with a possible special need. Parents are then able to model the encouragement shown to them and will be able to pass it on to their children. Confidence is the other overarching factor. This stems from having faith, trust, and belief in oneself. When parents are confident, they not only will get through the difficulties of raising children but will be equipped to take on the trials and tribulations of having a child who will need a lot of support. It is important to have these factors in order to increase identity, which will determine personal power.[5] When self-identity is strong, individuals realize their personal power and are able to pass it onto a new generation. When these two factors are lacking, there is a resultant decrease in awareness of value and personal power.

- Impact of the economy: These families are often single-parented (60.3% in Washington, DC) and headed by women.[5,6] They often live in low-income or subsidized housing and are likely receiving governmental assistance. The employment rate is low and when they are employed, it is often for minimal wages. In 2006 to 2007, this corresponded to 150% of poverty.[6] These economic factors affect the previously identified issues and serve to undergird the lack of resources, education, literacy, exposure, and the list goes on.
- Communication disorders are not life-threatening: Because individuals do not die from a communication disorder (with the exception of swallowing disorders), the need to follow-up on these services is not seen as a priority for some families. They fail to see that communication is the base for the quality of life and do not realize that if they do not communicate effectively, it will affect academic performance, social skills, and employment later in life.

The Need for Interprofessional Practice

As indicated, coordinating clinical services for urban families is quite the challenge, and the follow-up and carryover are often lost for a variety of the aforementioned reasons. One of the ways to combat this issue is through interprofessional practice. Interprofessional practice for an urban ACC is beneficial to this population for several reasons:

1. All professionals are involved in care simultaneously
2. There is increased communication with the patient
3. The professionals involved in the process can actually talk with each other right then and there
4. It decreases the lag time in services and allows the professional to touch base at the time of the visit.

The information that follows depicts the thoughts and processes used to establish an interprofessional practice in southeast Washington, DC, at an urban ACC. First, the current states of practice at the ACC and the Division of Hearing and Speech are described; then the model the authors envision for improving collaboration and coordination of care is reviewed.

CURRENT STATE OF PRACTICE
Ambulatory Care Center

Children's National Health System has demonstrated a long-standing commitment to provide comprehensive primary care services within the DC communities of greatest need. With the leases lapsing on two of its locations in small, outdated facilities in Southeast, DC, a decision was made to relocate and merge the two locations into a brand new, state-of-the art facility, the CHC-Anacostia.

Key features of the original sites included

- Located in Health Professional Shortage Areas as designated by US Department of Health and Human Services' Health Resources and Services Administration
- Certified as level 3 Patient-Centered Medical Homes by the National Committee for Quality Assurance
- Roughly 90% of the patients served in the two sites were publicly insured
- In fiscal year 2016 (July 2015–June 2016), the two sites combined conducted close to 24,000 patient visits
- See **Table 1** for a brief overview of the services provided in the original locations.

During the planning of the new CHA location, it was strategically determined that the larger facility presented an opportunity to provide space for rotating community health clinical programs to address conditions of high prevalence in the patients served (asthma, obesity, and mental health). Discussions were held with the Division of Hearing and Speech regarding the feasibility of incorporating an SLP into the clinical program rotation. Several factors were considered in the discussion including

- Demonstrated need: Based on claims data pulled from the fiscal year before the opening of the facility, there were almost 200 visits with a hearing and speech-related diagnosis for the three primary care sites in Southeast, DC. That visit count did not include patients who may carry a diagnosis that was not billed for during a primary care visit.
- Paucity of community resources: In DC, the EIP, also known as Strong Start, serves as a single point of entry for children presenting with developmental concerns. This program implements the Infants and Toddlers Program under the Individuals with Disabilities Education Act, Part C (34 CFR, Part 303). Children between the ages of birth and 3 years are automatically eligible to receive services if they have a diagnosis known to be associated with developmental delays. Children are also eligible if they demonstrate greater than 50% delay in any one of five developmental areas: cognitive, physical, communication, social, emotional, or adaptive. The DC public school system also provides assessments and interventions for those children deemed eligible to receive services between the ages of 2 years 8 months and 5 years 10 months through the Early Stages Center. This program serves children who attend DC public schools, are home-schooled, and those who have not yet entered the school system and live in DC. For children with mild delays who do not meet the threshold of eligibility for these programs, there are very few options for places to receive services in the East End, DC.

Inherent to an attempt to integrate the SLP into the CHA clinical rotation were several challenges:

- Scope of services: In a specialty-only outpatient setting, the SLP is responsible for identifying, coordinating, and executing treatment of children with concerns related to speech, language, stuttering, and voice, whether developmentally or neurologically based. This occurs in accordance with coordination of care between and among administration, physicians, and other specialty providers.
- Administrative challenges: Although both divisions involved in the integration are part of the same health system, they use different systems for electronic health record documentation and patient registration. Staff from the Division of Hearing and Speech uses Cerner, whereas those from General Pediatrics and Community Health use eClinicalWorks. The two systems are connected via an electronic hub that serves as a repository of documentation but they do not have interoperability.

Table 1
Description of preexisting services provided at Children's Health Center, Anacostia

Program Name	Program Description	Program Model or Staffing
Primary Care	Routine pediatric care from birth through age 21 with • Postpartum depression screening using the EPDS at ages 2 wk, 1, 2, 4, and 6 mo • Developmental screening using ASQ3 at ages 9, 18 and 30 mo • Autism screening using M-CHAT at ages 18 and 24 mo • Mental health screening using SDQ annually between ages 4 and 17 y	Team-based care model using pediatric health care provider paired 1–2:1 with an ambulatory patient care technician and 2–3:1 with a registered nurse or licensed practical nurse with ancillary support provided by social worker and health educator
Reach Out and Read	Incorporation of reading promotion into pediatric visit through the provision of free, new books at well-child visits between the ages of 6 mo, and 5 y with encouragement of parents to read aloud with their children	Book donations distributed by pediatric health care provider with anticipatory guidance
Psychology and Psychiatry	Colocated mental health providers for assessment and comanagement of behavioral health issues including brief psychotherapy and medication management	In-house direct referral and consultative services with pediatric management on stabilization in most cases
Healthy Families America	Intensive home visitation services conducted in partnership with the Mary's Center for Maternal and Child Health, a federally qualified health center for at-risk families, with enrollment during pregnancy through 3 mo of age	In-house and community-based referrals to a family support worker after assessment
Healthy Generations	Wraparound medical and case management services for parenting teens through and their children through age 21	Pediatric health care provider team Dedicated case management services provided by a social worker
Lactation Support Center	Integrated breastfeeding counseling, education, and support provided to families through the attainment of personal breastfeeding goal or 12 mo of age	In-house and community-based referrals to peer and professionally trained lactation support providers
Women, Infants, and Children Program (WIC)	Federally funded supplemental nutrition program for pregnant mothers and children through 5 y of age	In-house and community-based referrals to WIC nutritionists and technicians
Healthy Together	Medicolegal partnership with Children's Law Center to provide pro bono legal services for health-facing legal issues with special emphasis on medical access, housing, and educational placement issues	On-site Children's Law Center attorneys providing direct referral and consultative services Lobby education training sessions offered in conjunction with health educator

Abbreviations: EPDS, Edinburgh Postnatal Depression Scale; SDQ, Strengths and Difficulties Questionnaire.

Health care providers and social workers from the Division of General Pediatrics and Community Health are granted access to records in Cerner.

Speech-Language Pathology Services

The Hearing and Speech Division has been a part of Children's National Health System since an official merger of the Children's Hearing and Speech Center with the Children's National Health System back in the 1970s. The Children's Hearing and Speech Center sees more than 13,000 children each year in both speech-language pathology and audiology services, as well as inpatient and outpatient services. The center also provides services and lends support to a variety of teams throughout the institution. A list of the teams is presented in **Table 2**. To better understand the scope of services offered by the SLP, a modified depiction is presented in **Fig. 1**. This gives an idea of the depth and breadth of both the evaluation and treatment processes offered by the profession of speech-language pathology.

An Interprofessional Practice Model for an Urban Ambulatory Care Clinic

Table 3 provides an overview of how speech-language pathology fits into the everyday operation of the ACC. Every program has cause to offer speech and language services. It further explains what the services are and what staff is important for implementation.

Overarching principles

There are three overarching principles associated with this model depicted in **Fig. 2**. The principles of multicultural knowledge, professional clinical knowledge, and community knowledge are precursors to the clinical interaction and must be addressed by all service providers to make the clinical environment effective. An explanation for each is listed here.

Multicultural knowledge It is important for service providers to understand that in any clinical encounter culture is present. In this model, culture should be considered in its broadest sense and should go beyond race. Clinical service providers should be mindful that they bring their own culture to all clinical encounters, as do the patients and their families. Clashes occur when two cultures misunderstand each other. It is important to know as much about the attributes that contribute to culture as possible. Examples might include but are not limited to features such as language, dress, food preferences, customs, child rearing practices, values, beliefs, and lifestyle.

Table 2	
Current teams: Division of Hearing and Speech participation	
Speech-Language Pathology	**Audiology**
Cochlear implant	Cochlear implant
Center for Autism Spectrum Disorders	Center for autism spectrum disorders
Craniofacial	Craniofacial
Neurofibromatosis	Neurofibromatosis
Voice	ENT
Velopharyngeal incompetence	Cytomegalovirus
Aerodigestive	Oncology
Cardiology	
Modified barium swallow	
Feeding	
Alternative and augmentative communication	

Abbreviation: ENT, Ear, Nose and Throat

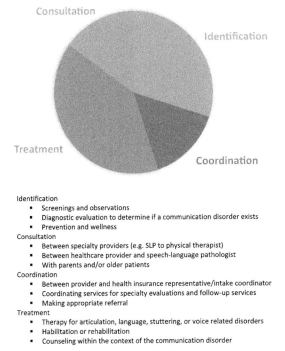

Identification
- Screenings and observations
- Diagnostic evaluation to determine if a communication disorder exists
- Prevention and wellness

Consultation
- Between specialty providers (e.g. SLP to physical therapist)
- Between healthcare provider and speech-language pathologist
- With parents and/or older patients

Coordination
- Between provider and health insurance representative/intake coordinator
- Coordinating services for specialty evaluations and follow-up services
- Making appropriate referral

Treatment
- Therapy for articulation, language, stuttering, or voice related disorders
- Habilitation or rehabilitation
- Counseling within the context of the communication disorder

Fig. 1. Scope of service for speech-language pathology.

The goal with culture is to strive for cultural competency (understanding other cultures) and cultural humility (self-reflection to better understand cultures). The idea is to get to the point at which culture becomes a natural part of clinical interactions so that no thought goes into how to interact with the patients or their families. When this happens, it is automatically done appropriately each time. This comes from making it conscious and deliberate initially, until it becomes second nature.

Community knowledge Community knowledge is different from cultural knowledge in that this area focuses on the specific environment, recognizing that a community can have a culture of its own. This, in some ways, becomes a subculture. With community knowledge in mind, it is important to know some of the following variables:

- What are the physical boundaries of the community?
- Who lives in the community?
- What might a typical family unit look like?
- Who are considered leaders in the community?
- How is medical support viewed in the community?
- What are some expectations of health care providers in the community?
- What might be considered a pitfall in the community?

To gather this information, health care providers and administrators might consider doing some of the following before opening a new facility or developing a model:

- Interview community leaders.
- Gather as much written information as possible from sources such as newspaper articles and magazines.

Table 3		
Description of ideal services infused with speech-language pathology		
Preexisting Program	**Speech-Language Pathology Infusion**	**Staffing**
Primary care	Same-day consultative services Scheduled evaluations Speech and language Prevention and wellness	Pediatric health care provider Nurse SLP Clinical operations representative
Reach Out and Read	Distribution of brochures for speech and language development at well-child visits Parent training sessions for language enrichment in the home	Pediatric health care provider SLP
Psychology and Psychiatry	Collaboration and coordination for referrals Use of children's telemedicine for virtual visits	Mental health provider Pediatric health care provider SLP Telemedicine liaison
Healthy Families America	Provide consultation as needed Provide prevention and wellness information to expectant parents	Home visitation staff SLP
Healthy Generations	Same-day consultative services or scheduled evaluations SLP enters in examination room with pediatric health care provider	Pediatric health care provider Nurse Social worker SLP
Lactation Support Center	Consultation when babies have difficulties feeding	Lactation specialist Pediatric health care provider SLP
WIC	Consultation with families about connection between nutrition and feeding or language development Participation in health fairs Prevention and wellness	WIC counselor SLP
Healthy Together	Consultation Advocacy and outreach	Law center attorney Health educator SLP

- Have conversations with historians to seek a perspective of the community.
- Visit churches and other religious organizations and schools to know the community.
- Observe people in highly trafficked areas of the community to understand the use of language and parent-children interactions.

Professional clinical knowledge This area deals with the health care service provider's fund of knowledge. It encompasses not only the university training she or he has had, but also how she or he has used it in a practical format to meet the needs of patients. Clinical knowledge should be ongoing and continuous to support new practice approaches.

Although this area is listed second in the model, it is purposefully discussed last in the principles. It is critical to understand that both cultural knowledge and community knowledge feed into and enhance the professional clinical knowledge. When service providers put all three of these components together, the combination strengthens the clinical encounter and lessens the possibility of medical errors.

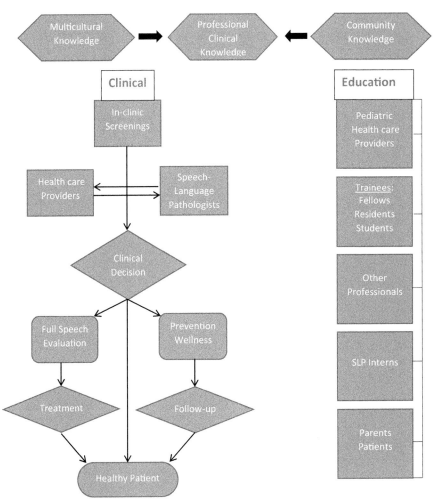

Fig. 2. Model for interprofessional practice.

Clinical

The model for interprofessional practice depicted in **Fig. 2** has several components that lend to the clinical coordination of patient care. This portion of the model is central to its success and all the components lead to this process.

In-clinic screenings This model supports the idea of the SLPs being in the examination room with the health care provider instead of the traditional way of waiting for a referral. As the health care provider is gathering information, the SLP is observing the patient, asking questions as well, administering screening tasks, discussing findings with the health care providers, and going over next steps with the parents and/or patients. This is very helpful when working with young children and older children or adolescents if they are new to the practice.

Health care providers and speech-language pathologists With this model, the health care providers are placed in the position of enhanced communication with each other. It becomes a 2-way street to continuous learning. The health care provider learns more about communication disorders and how to refer, and the SLP learns more about how the medical process works and how decisions are made.

Clinical decision During the course of discussion, a clinical decision is made about the patient regarding whether he or she needs the next phase of care. It is also a great opportunity to enhance the education and learning of trainees and other service providers. The advantage of this model is it moves quickly in both the clinical exchange and the decision-making processes. It is also a great model for identifying the children who are at high risk for a communication disorder.

Full speech-language evaluation If deemed appropriate, some children will need a full speech-language evaluation. This entails examining the following parameters in more detail:

- Receptive language
- Expressive language
- Pragmatic or social language
- Voice
- Speech fluency
- Articulation or phonology
- Oral structures and function
- Cognition screening
- Hearing screening.

Prevention and wellness In some cases, children might need support instead of a full speech-language evaluation. In those situations, the SLP will engage the parents and instruct them on how to monitor and/or facilitate speech-language skills at home. Educational information about speech and language disorders is shared with the parents so that they are encouraged to promote a healthy communication lifestyle.

Treatment Some children might need speech-language therapy after the results of the full evaluation are determined. This entails weekly sessions to address the deficient areas. Parental participation and pediatric health care provider awareness are very crucial to the results of treatment.

Follow-up Occasionally, patients are seen for follow-up screenings when there are questions about their communication performance or if screening results are inconclusive or just below the threshold of concern. The follow-up is done to assess progress in performance with the implementation of a home-based language enrichment plan.

Healthy patient The entire idea is to see a healthy patient with appropriate communication health.

Education

The model also has an education component. The education part of the model is both formal and informal. The informal portion occurs in the consultation portion of the in-clinic screening. It also occurs in preconferencing before seeing the patient or post-conferencing after seeing the patient. The formal part of the education process happens during staff meeting updates, in-service trainings, workshops, and invited presentations. Topics for discussion may include

- Normal speech and language development
- When and how to refer

- Stuttering
- Voice disorders
- Hearing health
- Autism spectrum disorders
- The roles and responsibilities of the SLP

These topics are modified and put in lay terms when using them for parent education workshops. This is a crucial part of the model because it overlaps with the clinical portion and serves to support the clinical activities.

SUMMARY

Now that the model the authors envision for interprofessional practice in the ACC is reviewed, we will summarize this discussion by revisiting the case of Z. Johnson to demonstrate how the course of her care could have been affected by such collaborative and coordinated care. Using the ideal model, Z. Johnson's parents would have received language enrichment education beginning at birth. This education would have better equipped them to identify red flags in language development to allow for earlier detection of her deviation from expected language acquisition. In this model, the SLP would have been present during the encounter at which the concern for her language delay was initially raised and would have conducted screenings to allow for prompt validation of this concern. On validation of the concern, Z. Johnson would have received a full speech evaluation by the SLP who would have also promptly scheduled an audiological evaluation. Delays in initiation and lapses in speech therapy services would have been avoided because there would be no need to transition between programs based on her aging out. Z. Johnson's primary care provider and parents would have not only received real-time progress reports but also ongoing education and training to support continued language development. It is likely that with earlier intervention, Z. Johnson could have entered preschool with age-appropriate speech and language skills. However, if additional services were needed, her SLP would have been available to assist with the development of an IEP to be carried out by her school. In this case, the SLP would have remained involved and in communication with her parents and health care provider to assess her progress and need for continued services until services were no longer deemed necessary.

REFERENCES

1. The National Academies Press. Speech and language disorders in children: Implications for the Social Security Administration's Supplemental Security Income program. In: Chapter 6 overall conclusions. 2016. Available at: https://www.nap.edu/read/21872/chapter/8. Accessed April 28, 2017.

2. McNeilly L. Rise in speech-language disorders in SSI-supported children reflects national trends. The ASHA Leader 2016. https://doi.org/10.1044/leader.PA2.21032016.np. 21 online only.

3. Matos A. Graduation rates to an all-time high at D.C. Public Schools. The Washington Post. 2016. Available at: https://www.washingtonpost.cm/local/education/graduation-rates-climb-again-as-dc-public-schools. Accessed May 1, 2017.

4. Harkness J. How poverty affects children's language skills. 2015. Available at: https://borgenporject.org/poverty-affects-childrens-language-skills/. Assessed April 28, 2017.

5. U.S. Department of Health and Human Services, Centers for Disease Control and Prevention. Available at: https://wwwn.cdc.gov/CommunityHealth/profile/currentprofile/DC/Washington/310044. Assessed May 1, 2017.
6. Reed J. Who is low-income in DC? DC Fiscal Policy Institute, October 26, 2010. Available at: http://www.dcfpi.org/who-is-low-income-in-dc. Assessed May 1, 2017.

The Future of Pediatric Speech-Language Pathology in a More Collaborative World

 CrossMark

Alan W. Dow, MD, MSHA[a],*, Carole K. Ivey, PhD, OTR/L[b], Brian B. Shulman, PhD, CCC-SLP, BCS-CL[c]

KEYWORDS

- Interprofessional practice • Interprofessional education
- Speech-language pathology • Networks • Teams

KEY POINTS

- Despite increasing emphasis on interprofessional practice, health care practitioners still primarily work in parallel rather than collaboratively and interdependently.
- Effective interprofessional practice depends not only on interpersonal determinants but also structural, regulatory, and governmental determinants that can be barriers or enablers to optimal collaboration.
- A major barrier to collaborative interprofessional practice is that care is often provided by different teams in different locations over time, a so-called network. Certain practitioners, including speech-language pathologists, are ideally positioned to bridge networks as boundary spanners, individuals who coordinate care across teams within a patient's network.
- To train practitioners to enhance interprofessional practice, students should receive interprofessional education as part of their professional programs. Practitioners need to engage in interprofessional continuing education relevant to their professional context, and leaders, researchers, and educators need to continue to refine models for a shared approach to practice.
- Done well, interprofessional practice can help health care practitioners reach their aspirations for higher quality, more equitable care.

Disclosure Statement: The authors have no commercial or financial conflicts of interest and no funding sources to disclose.

[a] Interprofessional Education and Collaborative Care, Virginia Commonwealth University, Box 980071, Richmond, VA 23298-0071, USA; [b] Department of Occupational Therapy, School of Allied Heatlh, Virginia Commonwealth University, Box 980008, Richmond, VA 23298-0008, USA; [c] Department of Speech-Language Pathology, School of Health and Medical Sciences, Seton Hall University, 400 South Orange Avenue, South Orange, NJ 07079, USA
* Corresponding author.
E-mail address: alan.dow@vcuhealth.org

This issue of *Pediatrics Clinics of North America* focuses on interprofessional practice through the lens of speech-language pathology. Interprofessional practice, as defined by the World Health Organization,[1] is when: "multiple health workers from different professional backgrounds provide comprehensive services by working with patients, their families, caregivers, and communities to deliver the highest quality of care across settings." The articles in this issue describe some successes in interprofessional practice, particularly for specific health conditions. However, they also highlight some of the challenges to optimal collaborative practice and identify some areas for future research and innovation in both education and care delivery.

THE LIMITATIONS OF TEAMWORK

Schreck and Golom[2] begin the issue with an overview of teamwork and interprofessional practice. In particular, they note several problems and challenges with the current state of teamwork in health care. First, they note that individuals often perceive more teamwork than truly exists. Rather than working in a collaborative fashion, groups of practitioners often work in parallel. Although they may perceive teamwork as they work in parallel with nearby colleagues, they do not realize the benefits of teamwork to themselves and their patients.

Drawing on the organizational development literature, they note 1 defining feature of teams is sharing a purpose and plan for work. In health care, the shared purpose is usually clear, improving the health of the patient. Yet, the plan for work is often not fully shared among team members. Critical questions teams in health care should be able to answer include

- How has each practitioner's plan for work evolved based on changes to the patient?
- How should that new individual plan interact with the updated plans of other health care practitioners?
- What expertise should be added to the new plan of care?
- What expertise should be subtracted in order to limit the complexity of the plan and the chance for error?

All of these questions are evidence of another defining feature of teamwork: interdependence. Team members embrace the reliance on each other, because it leads to a better overall outcome.

Why then is poor teamwork in health care implicated in so many problems and challenges faced by team members? Golom and Schreck provide some insight to this question. They note the ideal team size is between 5 and 6 members; team effectiveness decreases as the size of team increases beyond this range. Yet, the typical health care team is massive. A recent study looking at the number of health care practitioners involved in 2 months of cancer care for 100 patients showed the median team size was 117.[3] Not surprisingly, these teams are too large to be interdependent and to be able to develop a shared plan for work. Subsequent failures of desired interdependence then lead to poor outcomes.

How then should practitioners navigate these complex structures of work to best help patients, their families, and society? The remaining articles within this issue provide some hints on tackling these challenges.

NETWORKS AND BOUNDARY SPANNERS

First, health care practitioners should begin to think of health care as a network of teams. Although certain professional contexts have discrete teams with interdependence in plans of care, care typically passes between sets of teams as the patient's needs evolve. This arrangement of care has been called a network[4] or a multiteam system.[5] The practitioners who work in these networks and bridge these teams have been called boundary spanners or knowledge brokers.[6] These individuals must coordinate care between the different teams in order to ensure the safest, most effective care. Speech-language pathology often fills this essential role as a boundary spanner in networks. The following is an example.

Consider a child with chronic health problems including the need for the services of a speech-language pathologist. Like all children, the child has both medical and educational needs. In the medical arena, care is often led by a physician; however, physicians are rare in the educational setting. Meanwhile, in the educational arena, the instructional program is led by a teacher. But, teachers are rare in the medical setting. Certain professions, however, span both professional contexts (eg, speech-language pathology, occupational therapy, and nursing). Across these arenas, consistency of theoretic approach, assessment, and plan of care are critical for ensuring that the medical and educational plans are integrated and that the child thrives. In this responsibility, speech-language pathologists are leaders just as much as physicians or teachers are leaders in their specific domains. The speech-language pathologist leads, collaborates, and follows to create a stronger network of teams for the child.

Other articles in this issue focus on a specific disease state that exemplifies different arrangements of teamwork, networking, or both. Kummer's[7] review of the evaluation and treatment of cleft lip and palate describe an interprofessional team that leverages the expertise of multiple disciplines to collaborate with the patient and family on a plan of care. Seeking to be a truly interdependent team, these health care practitioners should meet collectively to review the patient's condition and plan the next steps in care.[8] These planning activities should continue iteratively as long as a team-based approach is needed.

Similarly, Lipner and Huron[9] illustrated how the neonatal intensive care unit (NICU) is an ideal setting for interprofessional teamwork. With patients, families, and practitioners colocated in the same setting, collaboration is supported by structures of care such as daily rounds. The structure of care is designed to engender collaboration and interdependence. However, this article also foreshadowed the challenges of transitioning between teams and networks by identifying the difficulties of handing off NICU graduates to a neurodevelopmental team to ensure ongoing evaluation and treatment after the NICU stay.

Contrast care in the NICU or of patients with cleft lip and palate has the imperative to evaluate late talkers[10] or in the broader realm of early intervention.[11] Here, practitioners, including the speech-language pathologist, who identify a concern must be a boundary spanner and activate the right part of the network to evaluate the issue and advance the child's best interest. Now, the individual practitioner is engaging the network, potentially to bring a team to bear on the health concern of the child. In addition, in both examples, the role of the health care professional is to liaise between patients and families, education, and health care.

Yet, being a boundary spanner is not simply about making connections; it is about judgment. In their review of the evaluation of feeding problems, Borowitz and Borowitz[12] noted that feeding problems are often benign, raising the question of when and if the interprofessional network should be activated to evaluate this concern. This is a fundamental challenge with networking; not only must practitioners know the network, they must know when to activate it and which part to activate. An analogous difficulty underlies Sedrak and Doss'[13] discussion of pediatric dental care. Although dental caries are the most common chronic disease in children, the shortage of dental practitioners highlights the need for all practitioners to be astute about when and how to refer to dental practitioners while also developing oral health expertise among nondental practitioners.

Working across a network is not only important for accessing care but also for ongoing management. Prelock and colleagues[14] describe the coaching in context model for children with autism spectrum disorder. In this article, the focus is not on evaluation but rather ongoing treatment and integration with the patient's life beyond the health setting. Spanning health care, education, and other social situations, the authors emphasize the tension between being patient- and family-centered while working across a diffuse network of professionals striving to help the patient.

Even in a setting that seems ripe for teamwork, barriers to interdependence persist. The evaluation of children with communication disorders requires collaboration among speech-language, psychological, and medical professionals.[15] Yet, synchronous care faces several barriers. Evaluations must be conducted over multiple days because of the impact of fatigue on the child's performance. Then, the team must meet face to face to develop a collaborative plan. Finally, once the team has completed the evaluation and developed the optimal plan, the plan must be discussed with the patient and family and implemented within the network of professionals, including educators, who will subsequently execute the plan of care. But, which individuals are best suited to counsel the patient initially? Who should be involved in follow-up? How will health care professionals work with teachers who do not share similar conceptual frameworks and are rarely located in the same place? This article captures why seemingly simple opportunities for collaboration become time consuming and frustrating.

THE MANY-LAYERED CHALLENGE OF INTERPROFESSIONAL PRACTICE

Underlying these challenges to interprofessional practice are important determinants of collaboration. With their discussion of otitis media, Welling and Ukstins[16] provide an incisive look at these determinants to interprofessional practice. Framing their article through the disciplinary lenses of both health care and education, they identify several categories of impediments to successful collaboration between these 2 professional contexts, including differences in conceptual frameworks, evaluation approaches, nomenclature, legal obligations, and reimbursement for services. The barriers and enablers to collaboration are not just interpersonal; they are often structural, regulatory, and governmental.[17] To practice more interprofessionally, leaders need to develop systems to lower these hurdles while practitioners continue to struggle to negotiate these obstacles to optimal collaboration.

TOWARD A MORE COLLABORATIVE WORLD

How then should health professionals proceed to achieve the goal of more collaborative health care? Many educators from across the health professions have taken important first steps by integrating interprofessional education into the curriculum for each degree-seeking profession. All such programs now have accreditation requirements that mandate interprofessional education[18] including speech-language pathology.[19] An example accreditation requirement for speech-language pathology graduate programs is to "understand how to perform effectively in different interprofessional team roles to plan and deliver care—centered on the individual served—that is safe, timely, efficient, effective, and equitable." This requirement underscores the role of the speech-language pathologist as a patient-centered care boundary spanner who engages in both teamwork and networking. The work before educators now is to determine how best to teach and assess these abilities.

Additionally, interprofessional practice is especially important for continuing education and practice-based interventions. Current practitioners, for the most part, have not partaken in interprofessional education in their degree programs and may need to catch up to current learners and the entering workforce. In addition, because teams and networks are often shaped by local context, interprofessional continuing education grounded in an individual's actual practice may be more impactful than the usual continuing education focused on updating core knowledge. Practice-focused, interprofessional continuing education may better help practitioners serve their patients within the existing structures of care.

Finally, interprofessional education must be paired with interventions that enable interprofessional practice. Of the beneficial interventions focused on enhancing interprofessional practice,[20] all have focused on improving the process of care through interventions such as structured meetings, redesigned medical rounds, checklists, or coaching. Although education and training were a part of some of these interventions, educational interventions alone have not been successful. Better interprofessional practice requires a supportive context. Importantly, a successful intervention in 1 context may not generalize to a different context. Clearly, changes in the approach to care are essential for practicing more interprofessionally, yet identifying which changes work best where and for which practitioners is a critical area for further research.[21]

Some overarching frameworks may be useful to guide interventions. For example, in this issue, McNeilly[22] provides an important example of an approach that can support more effective networking. The World Health Organization's International Classification of Functioning, Disability and Health (ICF) framework provides a common approach to understanding an individual's health conditions within the context of his or her life. In addition, it provides a method for tracking the impact of interventions on wellness. As a clinical process built on the foundation of patient-centered care, the ICF framework starts to address the limitations by supporting a shared model presented across a network.

Other articles in this issue also suggest models for enhanced interprofessional practice. Prelock and colleagues'[14] coaching in context model could be used as a shared framework for interprofessional interventions. Liu and colleagues[15] and Lipner and Huron[9] have begun to identify the barriers to the transition between teamwork and networking and some possible approaches to overcome the challenges in children with communication disorders and infants departing the NICU, respectively. Most notably, Welling and Ukstins[16] have begun to outline the parameters of a discussion around the structural barriers to interprofessional practice between educators and health care practitioners. These are all examples of areas that could drive research and innovation forward in the field.

ASPIRATIONS FOR A MORE COLLABORATIVE WORLD

The aspirations of better interprofessional education and collaborative practice are improved health outcomes, lower cost, enhanced patient experience, and increased practitioner satisfaction.[23] Robinson and colleagues[24] explain why better interprofessional practice has such potential, and why the speech-language pathology profession is critical to achieving these goals. Although many patients receive exceptional care in the United States, too many individuals still do not receive needed services. The gap between those who receive the best care and those who receive the least care is the biggest area for improvement in the US health care system. Robinson has described how speech-language pathologists can be the extension of the interprofessional team that reaches into the community to begin to solve the greatest challenge to health in the United States, health inequity.

As boundary spanners situated in both health care and community-based institutions like schools, speech-language pathologists are positioned to work directly with families. They can identify unmet needs early and close the gap between people who need health, social, or educational services and the networks that deliver these services. This is the aspiration of interprofessional practice, to better meet the needs of society as a whole. It just takes finding ways to work better together.

REFERENCES

1. World Health Oranization. Framework for action on interprofessional education and collaborative practice. Geneva (Switzerland): World Health Organization; 2010.
2. Schreck J, Golom F. The journey to interprofessional practice: are we there yet. Pediatr Clin North Am 2017.
3. Dow A, Zhu X, Sewell D, et al. Teamwork on the rocks: rethinking interprofessional practice as networking. J Interprof Care 2017;1–2 [Epub ahead of print].
4. Reeves S, Lewin S, Espin S, et al. Inteprofessional teamwork for health and social care. Oxford (United Kingdom): Blackwell; 2010.
5. Marks M, DeChurch L, Mathieu J, et al. Teamwork in multiteam systems. J Appl Psychol 2005;90(5):964–71.
6. Long J, Cunningham F, Braithwaite J. Bridges, brokers and boundary spanners in collaborative networks: a systematic review. BMC Health Serv Res 2013;13:158.
7. Kummer A. A pediatrician's guide to cleft palate speech and non-cleft causes of velopharyngeal insufficiency (VPi). Pediatr Clin North Am 2017.
8. Dow A, DiazGranados D, Mazmanian P, et al. Applying organizational science to health care: a framework for collaborative practice. Acad Med 2013;88(7):952–7.
9. Lipner H, Huron R. Developmental care of the pre-term infant: from NICU through high-risk infant follow-up. Pediatr Clin North Am 2017.
10. Capone Singleton N. Late talkers: why the 'wait and see' approach is outdated. Pediatr Clin North Am 2017.
11. Coufal K, Woods J. Interprofessional Collaborative Practice: what that means for early intervention service delivery. Pediatr Clin North Am 2017.
12. Borowitz K, Borowitz S. Feeding problems in infants and children: assessment and etiology. Pediatr Clin North Am 2017.
13. Doss L, Sedrak M. Open up and let us in: an interdisciplinary approach to oral health. Pediatr Clin North Am 2017.
14. Prelock P. Supporting children with autism and their families: a model for interprofessional practice. Pediatr Clin North Am 2017.
15. Liu L, Simms M, Zhart D. A multidisciplinary team approach to the differential diagnosis of children with communication disorders. Pediatr Clin North Am 2017.
16. Welling DR, Ukstins CA. Otitis media: beyond the examination room. Pediatr Clin North Am 2017;65(1):105–23.
17. Lawlis T, Anson J, Greenfield D. Barriers and enablers that influence sustainable interprofessional education: a literature review. J Interprof Care 2014;28(4):305–10.
18. Zorek J, Raehl C. Interprofessional education accrediting standards in the USA: a comparative analysis. J Interprof Care 2013;27(2):123–30.

19. Council on Academic Accreditation in Audiology and Speech-Language Pathology. 2017. Available at: http://caa.asha.org/wp-content/uploads/Accreditation-Standards-for-Graduate-Programs.pdf. Accessed September 27, 2017
20. Reeves S, Pelone F, Harrison R, et al. Interprofessional collaboration to improve professional practice and healthcare outcomes. Cochrane Database Syst Rev 2017;(6):CD000072.
21. Reeves S. The importance of realist synthesis for the interprofessional field. J Interprof Care 2015;29(1):1–2.
22. McNeilly L. Using the ICF framework to achieve interprofessional functional outcomes for young children: a speech-language pathology perspective. Pediatr Clin North Am 2017.
23. Earnest M, Brandt B. Aligning practice redesign and interprofessional education to advance triple aim outcomes. J Interprof Care 2014;28(6):497–500.
24. Robinson T, Anderson D, Long S. The role of the speech-language pathologist in creating a model for interprofessional practice in an ambulatory care clinic. Pediatr Clin North Am 2017.

Moving?

Make sure your subscription moves with you!

To notify us of your new address, find your **Clinics Account Number** (located on your mailing label above your name), and contact customer service at:

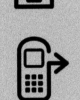

Email: **journalscustomerservice-usa@elsevier.com**

800-654-2452 (subscribers in the U.S. & Canada)
314-447-8871 (subscribers outside of the U.S. & Canada)

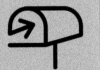

Fax number: **314-447-8029**

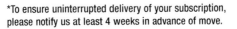

Elsevier Health Sciences Division
Subscription Customer Service
3251 Riverport Lane
Maryland Heights, MO 63043

*To ensure uninterrupted delivery of your subscription, please notify us at least 4 weeks in advance of move.

ELSEVIER